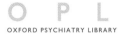

OXFORD PSYCHIATRY LIBRARY

Suicide Prevention

O P L

OXFORD PSYCHIATRY LIBRARY

Suicide Prevention

Robert D. Goldney,
MD, FRCPsych, FRANZCP

Professor and Head,
Discipline of Psychiatry,
University of Adelaide,
Australia

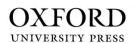

OXFORD
UNIVERSITY PRESS

OXFORD
UNIVERSITY PRESS

Great Clarendon Street, Oxford OX2 6DP

Oxford University Press is a department of the University of Oxford.
It furthers the University's objective of excellence in research, scholarship,
and education by publishing worldwide in

Oxford New York

Auckland Cape Town Dar es Salaam Hong Kong Karachi
Kuala Lumpur Madrid Melbourne Mexico City Nairobi
New Delhi Shanghai Taipei Toronto

With offices in

Argentina Austria Brazil Chile Czech Republic France Greece
Guatemala Hungary Italy Japan Poland Portugal Singapore
South Korea Switzerland Thailand Turkey Ukraine Vietnam

Oxford is a registered trade mark of Oxford University Press
in the UK and in certain other countries

Published in the United States
by Oxford University Press Inc., New York

British Library Cataloguing in Publication Data

Data available

Library of Congress Cataloging in Publication Data

Data available

Typeset by Newgen Imaging Systems (P) Ltd., Chennai, India
Printed in Italy
on acid-free paper by
L.E.G.O. S.p.A – Lavis TN

ISBN 978–0–19–953325–1

10 9 8 7 6 5 4 3 2 1

Whilst every effort has been made to ensure that the contents of this book are as
complete, accurate and-up-to-date as possible at the date of writing. Oxford
University Press is not able to give any guarantee or assurance that such is the case
Readers are urged to take appropriately qualified medical advice in all cases. The
information in this book is intended to be useful to the general reader, but should
not be used as a means of self-diagnosis or for the prescription of medication.

Contents

Preface

Suicide and suicidal behaviour evoke strong feelings. That is so not only for those directly affected—the individual, family, and friends, but also for potential therapists and the community at large.

Opinions about suicidal behaviour abound. That is not unexpected, as a number of different disciplines can reasonably offer their own perspective. That makes it particularly challenging to integrate data from diverse sources into a cohesive approach to suicide prevention at the individual level. In fact, it has led some to be unduly pessimistic.

Much is known about the contributing factors to suicide. Many observations from over a century ago have been confirmed by sophisticated research methodologies, and intervention programmes have been demonstrated to be effective. It is also important that the biological/mental disorder versus sociological/psychosocial influences dichotomy has increasingly been laid to rest.

Inevitably there will be areas in this book where my interpretation of the available data or opinion will not be shared by all. However, the aim of this pocketbook has been to integrate the best available research, with an acknowledgement of its limitation, in a practical and pragmatic approach to suicide prevention.

Robert Goldney,
April 2008
University of Adelaide,
Australia

Acknowledgements

Stimulating interaction with clinicians, researchers and volunteers from many Disciplines has been of inestimable value in refining both my clinical practice and my interpretation of the literature. Professor Johan Schioldann and Dr Sheila Clark contributed to earlier publications on the history of suicide prevention and bereavement after suicide respectively, which formed the basis for the relevant chapters in this book. The permission of Elsevier Limited to reprint Figure 7.1 from 'A novel integrated knowledge explanation of factors leading to suicide', published first in New Ideas in Psychology, 2003, 21:141–146, is also acknowledged. Finally, the willing assistance of the Commissioning Editor, Mr Peter Stevenson, and Assistant Commissioning Editor, Ms Emma Marchant, as well as that of my secretary, Ms Roslyn Mitchell, has been fully appreciated.

Symbols and abbreviations

BMI	body mass index
CATIE	Clinical Antipsychotic Trials of Intervention Effectiveness
CBT	Cognitive Behaviour Therapy
CSF	cerebrospinal fluid
DBT	Dialectical Behaviour Therapy
DST	dexamethasone suppression test
IASP	International Association for Suicide Prevention
IASR	International Academy of Suicide Research
IFOTES	International Federation of Telephonic Emergency Services
IPT	Interpersonal Therapy
MBCT	Mindfulness Based Cognitive Therapy
PAR	population attributable risk
RCT	randomized controlled trials
SMR	standardized mortality ratio
SSRI	selective serotonin re-uptake inhibitor
WHO	World Health Orgainsation

Chapter 1

Historical review

Key points

- Suicide has been documented since antiquity
- Contemporaneously relevant research has been conducted for over 200 years
- Many of the accepted social and mental disorder antecedents of suicide were well documented by the late 19th century.

1.1 Introduction

Although clinicians and researchers acknowledge that suicide has been written about since antiquity, in their day to day work they tend to ignore publications from previous decades, let alone those from over 100 years ago. This has led to the recent integration of psychosocial and biological factors in our understanding of suicidal behaviours being regarded as an advance on the predominant 20th century focus on psychosocial issues, which flowed from the influential late 19th century sociologist, Durkheim. Indeed, the casual observer could be forgiven for believing that there had not been any suicide research before Durkheim, let alone any which had addressed mental disorders and their inter-relationship with society. That is not the case.

1.2 Initial English reports

Suicide was documented and commented upon in Ancient texts, but John Sym's 1637 'Life Preservative Against Self-Killing Or, An Useful Treatise Concerning Life and Self-murder' was probably the first book in English to address suicide. Sym noted perceptively that 'Self-murder is prevented, not so much by arguments against the fact; which disswades from the conclusion; as by the discovery and removal of the motives and causes, whereupon they are tempted to do the same; as diseases are cured by removing of the causes, rather than of their symptoms.'

The next century was marked by European work until 1790, when Charles Moore wrote 'A Full Inquiry into the Subject of Suicide' in two volumes. He described the association between alcohol and suicide; the hereditary nature of some suicides; and he questioned the validity of suicide statistics. He also noted 'that there is a sort of madness in 'every' act of suicide, even when all idea of lunacy is excluded', and for those who work in the forensic/legal setting and have to determine the state of mind of those who have died by suicide, his comment that 'Such distinctions of sanity and insanity are too fine spin to be just or equitable' is particularly pertinent. Indeed, it is doubtful if anyone in the subsequent two hundred years has described that challenge more elegantly.

Box 1.1 Moore, 1790

- 'A sort of madness' in all suicide
- Difficulty in distinguishing sane and insane suicides
- Association of alcohol and gambling noted
- Some suicides inherited
- Validity of statistics questioned.

1.3 Early 19th century influences

There were significant changes in public attitudes to suicide in the first few decades of the 19th century. In England this was associated with the suicide in 1822 of Lord Castlereagh. He had been an influential and successful politician, whose suicide was probably associated with a melancholic illness. He was not denied a funeral, as should have been the case, and that led to considerable public debate. This was given further impetus in 1823, when a 22-year-old law student, Abel Griffiths, died by suicide and had the ignominy of being the last person to be buried at a cross roads. The rescinding of the law in regard to the treatment of the corpse of a suicide occurred soon after.

The initial medical model of suicide has been attributed primarily to the early 19th century French physician Esquirol (1821), although it is evident that he freely acknowledged the role of social factors as well. A similar broad approach was offered by Burrows in England, who in 1828 noted that suicide was 'a feature of melancholia', although he added that 'a doubt may naturally arise, whether it be not sometimes perpetrated by a sane mind'. He also referred to the relationship of homicide and infanticide to suicide; the possibility that suicide was 'sometimes innate or hereditary'; that suicide occurred in children; and that contagion could influence suicide. He stated that 'The medical treatment of the propensity to suicide, whether prophylactic or therapeutic, differs not from that which is applicable in cases of ordinary insanity', a comment reminiscent of Sym in 1637, and still pertinent today.

Social factors were also considered by other early commentators, including Karl Marx, who in 1846 introduced German scholars to the memoirs of Peuchet, the archivist of the Paris Prefecture of Police, who in 1838 had referred to suicide as a 'deficient organisation of our society'. Similarly, the mid-19th century Norwegian theologian and social researcher Eilert Sundt noted that 'if there is responsibility then it does not only rest on the individual who committed the act, but also on society'.

There was significant French work in the 1850s, including that of Lisle who in 1856 reviewed over 52,000 suicides, citing 48 causes including insanity, debt, gambling, and 'disappointed love'. Also in 1856, Brierre de Boismont reported on over 4,000 suicides, with no fewer than 18 broad causes. The extent of French contributions to mid-19th century suicide research can be gauged by noting that bibliographies of the prestigious Annales Médico-Psychologiques contain references to 138 papers addressing suicide between 1843 and 1878.

> **Box 1.2 Mid-19th century knowledge**
> - Importance of insanity in general noted
> - Melancholia and alcohol specifically referred to
> - Influence of societal organisation discussed
> - Interpersonal issues such as 'disappointed love' and 'reversal of fortune' noted
> - First classifications of suicide emerged.

In 1858 Bucknill and Tuke published what was to become the standard textbook of English psychiatry for many years. It contained a classification of three main types of suicide, with it arising from suicidal monomania, melancholia, or delusions and hallucinations. There was also a fourth type where 'it must obviously be very difficult to determine, in such cases, whether the individual was, or was not, a free agent at the time'.

It is doubtful whether there were any significant books devoted solely to suicide published in the United States in the 19th century, but there were research reports and commentaries, including those in the American Journal of Insanity, the forerunner to the American Journal of Psychiatry. In the first issue in 1844 the Editor, Brigham, commented on the probable under-reporting of suicides, and he also made the often quoted comment in regard to media publicity: 'That suicides are alarmingly frequent in this country is evident to all—and as a means of prevention, we respectfully suggest the propriety of not publishing the details of such occurrences'.

1.4 Late 19th century research

The Italian Morselli published his book 'Suicide: an Essay on Comparative Moral Statistics' in 1879 and by 1881 it had been translated into English and German. It is encyclopaedic in content, and arguably the most important work of 19th century suicidology. Westcott referred to it as a 'thoroughly scientific statistical work', although he added that it was 'hardly a readable book, consisting almost entirely of statistics …', and Tuke referred to it as a 'laborious work for a mass of information.' It contains detailed statistics, focusing on Italy, but also including data from a number of other countries. Individual sections of the book included 'Increase and regularity of suicide in civilised countries'; 'Social Influences'; 'Influences arising out of the biological and social conditions of the individual'; 'Individual psychological influences'; and 'Methods and places of Suicide'; before he provided a 'Synthesis' on the 'Nature and Therapeutics of Suicide'.

Morselli analysed age and suicide in different countries; education and suicide rates; and the 'Relation of Madness with Suicide', with the latter demonstrating an association between rates of 'mad people' and suicide. He also provided a perceptive view of emotional or psychic pain, noting that: 'it is a gross tautological sophism to give the title of 'moral suffering' to sorrow for a misfortune, to misery, privation, crossed love or jealousy, whilst they reserve the title of 'physical suffering' to pain which arises from a mechanical injury, from an irritation of the peripheral nerves, or disease of the intestines. The cause is unequal, but the effect is the same … the expression of moral suffering is the same as that of physical suffering'.

A less statistically burdened work than that of Morselli was provided by Westcott in 1885 in his book: 'Suicide: its History, Literature, Jurisprudence, Causation and Prevention'. He addressed the rates and means of suicide; its causes; the effect of urban and rural life; the influence of mental disease; suicide from imitation; and the effects of physical illness and hereditary factors. He even included a chapter on suicide in animals, a surprisingly contemporary set of observations in view of recent ethological conceptualizations of suicide.

Westcott was well aware of the importance of social issues, as in his preface he wrote: 'The question (of suicide) is one well worthy of the earnest consideration of the community; indeed, it may be legitimately regarded as one of our Social Problems, as it involves matters which are intimately connected with our social organisation, and is with propriety embraced in our legislative enactments'. It is also of interest, bearing in mind the concerns of some contemporary clinicians, that he observed 'now that a study of suicide as a fact has been instituted, it has fallen almost entirely into a statistical groove, to the neglect of research into the mental state and emotions of the unfortunate individuals who become victims'.

In 1892 there were comprehensive reviews of suicide research by Tuke and Savage in 'Tuke's Dictionary of Psychological Medicine'. Tuke presented an erudite historical perspective of suicide, noting that 'there has been no period in authentic history in which, so far as we know, there has been immunity from the practice of self destruction.' He referred to biblical suicides and then to Greek and Roman perspectives, before noting how attitudes gradually changed over the centuries. His epidemiological review was predominantly of European countries, although data from the United States and Australia were also presented.

Tuke had a critical appreciation of the limitations of some previous research. This is well illustrated in relation to those theories about suicidigenous areas and claims that suicide rates were related to geological formations or the weather. Thus Tuke stated that 'we confess that we accept the conclusions with considerable reserve, first, because the returns of suicide in different countries may differ in their completeness, and therefore may be misleading; and secondly, because the elements of the problem are so exceedingly complex that we are in great danger of referring a maximum amount of suicide to the wrong cause.' Such comments are no less pertinent today than when written by Tuke over 100 years ago.

Many of Tuke's observations have stood the test of time and subsequent research. The male-to-female preponderance of suicide is virtually identical to that found today; it is still the case that 'there is no doubt that agricultural distress increases the number of suicides'; similarly 'it would seem that divorce exercises a more injurious influence on the male than on the female sex'; there is a higher rate of suicide among doctors; suicide remains a reality in children; it is still true that 'the influence of imprisonment on the tendency to suicide … (is) well marked, especially in prisoners under 30 years of age'; as is the fact that 'the influence of alcohol or beer in the pro-duction of suicide is not disputed'; and it is also recognized that examples of hereditary suicide have occurred.'

Box 1.3 Contemporary relevance of late 19th century research

- Male to female ratio similar
- Importance of melancholia
- Alcohol influence
- Suicide occurs in children
- Role of contagion noted
- Effect of divorce, rural distress and prison
- Role of inherited factors acknowledged
- High suicide rate in doctors
- Communication component described
- Noted that self-mutilation provided relief
- Tension between statistical research as opposed to focussing on the individual
- Risk/benefit issues of management discussed.

Savage provided what could be interpreted as a surprisingly contemporary view of mental disorders and suicide. He acknowledged that suicide could occur with 'no other signs of insanity', and he also noted that 'In some cases of slight emotional disorder there may be an intention to pretend to commit suicide', a formulation which antedated the concept of the 'Cry for help' by seventy years. He observed that self-mutilation was performed in order to give relief; that 'All melancholic patients must be considered suicidal till they are fully known;' that even 'Simple melancholia of very slight depth is a very common cause of suicide;' and that 'Waves of depression occur in many neurotic but otherwise sane people, which often lead to suicide'. He also stated that 'Voices may command', and 'misery produced by constant occurrence of hallucinations, may act like constant pain.'

Savage wrote perceptively that in clinical management 'some risk must be run sooner or later, and it is necessary in curable cases to recognise that the too constant presentation of the idea of distrust to the patient's mind keeps up the morbidly suicidal state', an excellent description of the dilemma facing clinicians treating those who are suicidal.

Savage's work is also notable for his categorization of suicide. He observed that suicide could be either impulsive or deliberate, and the deliberate suicides included those with 'egotistical' and 'altruistic feelings.' In fact these terms had also been documented elsewhere as early as 1880, albeit without any subsequent attribution by Durkheim, who in 1897 described egoistic, altruistic, anomic, and fatalistic suicide, with the focus being on the predominance of societal influences on suicide.

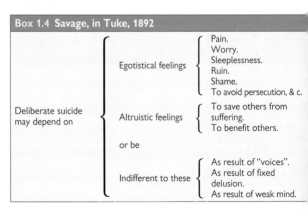

Box 1.4 Savage, in Tuke, 1892

Deliberate suicide may depend on	Egotistical feelings	Pain. Worry. Sleeplessness. Ruin. Shame. To avoid persecution, & c.
	Altruistic feelings	To save others from suffering. To benefit others.
	or be	
	Indifferent to these	As result of "voices". As result of fixed delusion. As result of weak mind.

1.5 **Conclusion**

This historical review illustrates the breadth and depth of enquiry about suicide which existed prior to the twentieth century. It is evident that increasingly during the 18th and 19th centuries the initial writings of theologians gave way to the more contemporary view of suicide being influenced not only by broad social issues, but also by factors such as mental disorders, the media, and occupation, and even the hereditary predisposition to suicide had been canvassed. In addition, there was an awareness of the limitations of the data and the challenges involved in drawing definitive conclusions in this area.

There had also been a demystification of earlier often punitive religious views, with the gathering of empirical data, so much so that there was a reaction to that, as illustrated by Westcott's comment in 1885 that suicide research had 'fallen almost entirely into a statistical groove'. That suggests that the ground was fertile for the subsequent sociological views of Durkheim and the emerging influence of psycho-analysis, both of which provided a counter to much of the earlier work, so much so that it has often been overlooked. However, it is no exaggeration to state that many of the findings of early researchers remain relevant today, and warrant greater recognition.

Key references

Goldney, R.D., Schioldann, J.A. (2000). Pre-Durkheim Suicidology, *Crisis*, **21**: 181–6.

Moore. C. (1790). A Full Inquiry Into The Subject Of Suicide etc. (2 vols). London: J. F. & C. Rivington.

Morselli, E. (1879). Il Suicidio. Saggio di statistica morale comparata. Milano: Dumolard. Vol. 21 of The 'Biblioteca Scientifica Internazionale'.—Idem (1881). Suicide. An Essay On Comparative Moral Statistics. Revised and Abridged By The Author For The English Version. London: C. Kegan Paul.

Tuke, D.H. (1892). A Dictionary of Psychological Medicine. London: J. & A. Churchill.

van Hoof, A.J. (1993). Suicide and parasuicide in ancient personal testimonies. *Crisis*. **14**, 76–82.

Westcott, W.W. (1885). A Social Science Treatise. Suicide, Its History, Literature, Jurisprudence, Causation and Prevention. London: H.K. Lewis.

Whitt, H.P. (2006). Durkheim's precedence in the use of the terms Egoistic and Altruistic Suicide: An Addendum. *Suicide Life Threat. Behav.*, **36**, 125–7.

Chapter 2

Definitions

> **Key points**
>
> - There are no universally agreed definitions of suicidal behaviour
> - There has been a plethora of terms attempting to accommodate the semantics and diversity of suicidal behaviour
> - A pragmatic approach based on suicidal intent and physical lethality is of most clinical utility.

2.1 Early nomenclature

For well over 100 years the nomenclature and classification of suicidal behaviour has defied general consensus. Forty years ago the World Health Organisation categorized theorists of suicidal behaviour into the Unitarians, for those who saw each attempt as an expression of wishing to die; the Binarians, who saw two groups, those who wished to die by their action and those who had not intended to die; the Pluralists, who saw various intentions in each attempt; and the Individualists, who saw each attempt as a unique situation.

There also arose a variety of terms seeking to clarify suicidal behaviours including gestures, ambivalent and serious; intentioned, sub-intentioned, un-intentioned and contra-intentioned cessation; and an early statistical typology delineated a depressed alienated group with high lethality, an angry alienated group whose behaviour was manipulative, and a heterogeneous third group with no specific characteristics. Attempted suicide was also referred to in diverse ways, including pseudocide, para-suicide, acute poisoning, self-injury, and deliberate self-harm.

2.2 Recent reviews

Since then there has been a plethora of terms for various aspects of suicidality, and a recent review described nine synonyms for suicidal ideation; nine for suicidal intent; ten for suicide threat or gesture; 36 for suicide attempt; and even 27 for suicide per se!

Such industry in defining the individual behaviour has been reflected in classifications of increasing complexity, resulting in complicated matrices with as many as 27 different categories. It is arguable whether these developments are of any practical use, although they may be of value from the research point of view. For the clinician, what appears to be of most importance is to determine what the antecedents of the suicidal behaviour may have been, no matter how it is defined.

It is apparent that many of the synonyms and categories embody several different concepts, often combined. Some refer purely to the semantics of attempted suicide, and others to clinical inferences of suicidal intent and physical lethality. Inevitably, some have assumed a pejorative quality.

2.3 **The wish to live and the wish to die**

Although one of the aims of this expanding nomenclature has been to acknowledge that persons who engage in suicidal behaviour may not have definitely wished to kill themselves, it sometimes appears that any component of wishing to die is minimized. The mixed feelings of wishing to live and wishing to die, the 'Janus face' of attempted suicide, have long been recognized, and experienced clinicians are well aware of both the expression of wanting to escape from an intolerable situation with little thought of death *per* se, as well as the generally observed feelings of relief of the survivors of potentially lethal suicidal acts.

It is probable that the very dichotomy of those who die and those who survive may have obscured the mixed feelings of these persons. The overlapping nature of those who die or survive has been long emphasized, and the distinction between them is not as clear-cut as is sometimes portrayed, as the most powerful predictor of suicide is previous suicidal behaviour, no matter how it is defined. For example, single emergency room visits for an overdose, suicidal ideation or self-harm are each strongly associated with subsequent suicide.

2.4 **An ethological approach**

Rather than attempting to introduce an artificial certainty into such nomenclatures, it is more logical to accept that suicidal behaviours are simply relatively non-specific responses to a wide variety of stimuli and mediators. This is consistent with an ethological conceptualization of suicidal behaviour, with the communication aspect, the 'cry for help', acting as an innate release mechanism, eliciting care from others. If the suicidal or care-eliciting behaviour is seen to be manipulative, or in ethologic terms cheating, then rejection or, at the very least ambivalence is the response of the potential carer. These are simply basic observations of what actually occurs.

There appear to be clinical advantages in adopting an observational or ethological conceptualization of suicidal behaviour. By accepting such acts as examples of relatively undifferentiated responses to stress, cognizance is taken of the environment, the person, and a variability of response, with mixed motivations and feelings. Such a formulation more readily allows a non-judgmental approach to the patient, with acceptance of both the appeal and wish to die components. In addition, it offers clarification of the nosological debate, rendering the differences more apparent than real.

2.5 **Pragmatic definitions**

The debate about the nosology of suicidal behaviour could be pursued ad infinitum, without satisfying all. It is pragmatic to assume that it involves a spectrum in terms of the individual's suicidal intent or wish to die, and the degree of lethality or physical threat to life. The term 'suicidality' embraces all of these aspects, and within suicidality there are four broad clinical categories:

- **Suicide**—a self-inflicted act resulting in death, albeit with varying suicidal intent
- **Attempted suicide**—self-injurious behaviour with varying degrees of suicidal intent and lethality
- **Suicidal ideation**—thoughts of self-injurious behaviour with variable suicidal intent but no lethality
- **Self harm**—deliberate non-fatal self injury with no suicidal intent.

Such simple definitions will not find favour with those who have assiduously pursued complex classifications in an attempt to accommodate widely variable degrees of suicidal intent and lethality in a scientifically rigorous manner. However, they are easily understood; they are unambiguous; they have stood the test of time; and, importantly, they allow for clinical judgement to be exercised in the individual suicidal person.

Notwithstanding these comments, in deference to those authors with strong views on the subject, their synonyms will be retained when referring to their specific studies. However, these pragmatic definitions will be used elsewhere.

Box 2.1 Suicidal intent and lethality associated with definitions of suicidal behaviour		
	Suicidal intent	*Lethality*
Suicide	Variable, usually high	Absolute
Attempted suicide	Variable	Variable
Suicidal ideation	Variable	Nil
Self-harm	Nil	Variable, usually low

2.6 **Other self-destructive behaviours**

It will be evident that no mention has been made of behaviour such as chronic self-defeating substance abuse or lack of compliance with treatments for potentially fatal physical illness. Whether such persons fall under the broad rubric of engaging in suicidal behaviour is open to debate. If one wished to include them, then the same broad principles of assessment and management that will be addressed would apply.

References

Crandall, C., Fullerton-Gleason, L., Aguero, R., La Valley, J. (2006). Subsequent suicide mortality among emergency department patients seen for suicidal behavior. *Acad. Emerg. Med.,* **13**, 435–42.

De Leo, D., Burgis, S., Bertolote, J.M., *et al.* (2006). Definitions of Suicidal Behavior. *Crisis*, **27**, 4–15.

Goldney, R.D. (2000). Ethology and Suicidal Behaviour. In K. Hawton, K. van Heeringen, eds. The International Handbook of Suicide and Attempted Suicide, 95–106. John Wiley & Sons Ltd., Chichester.

Haw, C., Bergen, H., Casey, D., Hawton, K. (2007). Repetition of deliberate self-harm: a study of the characteristics and subsequent deaths in patients presenting to a general hospital according to extent of repetition. *Suicide Life-Threat. Behav.*, **37**, 379–96.

Henderson, A.S., Hartigan, J., Davidson, J. *et al.* (1977). A Typology of Parasuicide. *Br. J. Psychiat.*, **131**, 631–41.

O'Carroll, P.W., Berman, A.L., Maris, R.W. *et al.* (1996). Beyond the Tower of Babel: A Nomenclature for Suicidology. *Suicide Life-Threat. Behav.*, **26**, 237–52.

Shneidman, E.S. (1985). Definitions of Suicide. John Wiley & Sons, New York.

Silverman, M.M. (2006). The language of suicidology. *Suicide Life-Threat. Behav.*, **36**, 519–32.

Silverman, M.M., Berman, A.L., Sanddal, (2007). Rebuilding the Tower of Babel: a revised nomenclature for the study of suicide and suicidal behaviors Part 2: Suicide—Related Ideation, Communications, and Behaviors. *Suicide Life-Threat. Behav.*, **37**, 264–77.

Chapter 3

Epidemiology

> **Key points**
>
> - About one million people die by suicide each year
> - Ten to twenty times that number attempt suicide
> - Suicide numbers are probably under-reported
> - There is wide variation of suicide rates both between and within countries
> - Suicide has increased in younger males in developed countries
> - Attempted suicide, suicidal ideation and self-harm have widely varying rates, but they share common antecedents
> - Findings from epidemiological data cannot necessarily be extrapolated to the individual person.

3.1 **The global suicide rate**

The World Health Organisation (WHO) has estimated that approximately one million people die each year by suicide, representing a global suicide rate of about 16 per 100,000. More people die by suicide each year than in wars, and in some countries the numbers are greater than deaths from motor vehicle accidents.

The difficulty of establishing reliable epidemiological data on suicide has been noted for over 200 years. The current WHO estimate is appreciably higher than the ten per 100,000 reported when data were first gathered by the WHO in 1950, but it is doubtful whether this represents a true increase. Only 21 countries reported suicide rates in 1950, and even by 1995 only 105 of more than 200 countries participated in WHO collation of data. The increase overall may also be accounted for by the recent inclusion of Northern and Eastern European countries with high rates.

3.2 **Under-reporting**

It is generally acknowledged that there is an under-reporting of suicide to a varying degree in different societies. However, the under-reporting is probably relatively constant between countries, or indeed between different regions in the same country, albeit with gradual change with, for example, a country's degree of religious affiliation, or changes in suicide ascertainment procedures. Whilst it is reasonable to compare suicide rates, due caution must be exercised because of such factors. High suicide rates are generally considered to be credible, with the caveat that rates can be artificially inflated if a country has a low population, where sporadic suicides can dramatically increase numbers per 100,000. On the other hand, very low rates are questionable as not only data gathering may be suspect, but religious and political imperatives may preclude reporting.

3.3 Diversity of suicide rates

The most recently available suicide statistics from a number of different countries demonstrate high rates in the Baltic States and countries of the Russian Federation, as well as in countries such as Japan. Low rates are reported from some Mediterranean countries and there are even lower rates elsewhere in the world, but those statistics are suspect.

There can be marked differences in suicide rates even within a relatively small geographical area, such as the eight-fold difference between Greece (3.4 per 100,000) and Slovenia (28.1 per 100,000). There can also be marked differences in the same country, as illustrated by the United States, where there is a three-fold variation between the low rates of the North Eastern states of New York and Massachusetts (about 6.5 per 100,000) compared to the mid West States of Montana and Nevada (about 19 per 100,000). There is a tendency for suicide to be more common in rural than urban areas, and that is particularly evident in China.

There are also marked differences between some ethnic groups, as demonstrated by African Americans having a lower rate (7 per 100,000) compared with white Americans (13.1 per 100,000). On the other hand, increased rates in Canadian Inuit, New Zealand Maori and Australian Aborigines have been reported. Such variations could not be related to the differing prevalence of mental disorders per se, and they emphasize the importance of psycho-social factors.

Table 3.1 provides suicide rates from a number of selected countries. It will be seen that data are not available for the same time periods for each country, making comparisons less reliable. In most countries suicide is more common in males, with the exception of rural China, where females predominate. Because of the large populations of China and India, suicide in those countries represents about 30% of suicides world-wide.

Table 3.1 Suicide rates per 100,000 for selected countries

Country (year)	Total	Men	Women
Lithuania (2005)	38.6	68.1	12.9
Belarus (2003)	35.1	63.3	10.3
Russia Fed (2004)	34.3	61.6	10.7
Slovenia (2003)	28.1	45.0	12.0
Hungary (2003)	27.7	44.9	12.0
Japan (2003)	25.5	38.0	13.5
Latvia (2004)	24.3	42.9	8.5
Sri Lanka (2005)	24.1	37.3	9.7
Ukraine (2004)	23.8	43.0	7.3
China (1999) Rural[1]	22.5	20.4	24.7
Belgium (1997)	21.1	31.2	11.4
Finland (2004)	20.3	31.7	9.4
Switzerland (2002)	19.8	27.4	12.5
France (2002)	17.8	26.6	9.5
Poland (2003)	15.3	26.7	4.5
Denmark (2001)	13.6	19.2	8.1
Sweden (2002)	13.2	19.5	7.1
New Zealand (2005)	13.1	20.1	6.4
Germany (2004)	13.0	19.7	6.6
Canada (2002)	11.6	18.3	5.0
Ireland (2002)	11.5	18.9	4.1
Norway (2004)	11.5	15.8	7.3
United States (2004)	11.1	17.7	4.6
Portugal (2003)	11.0	17.5	4.9
India (2002)	10.5	12.8	8.0
Australia (2005)	10.3	16.4	4.3
Netherlands (2004)	9.3	12.7	6.0
Iceland(2003)	9.0	13.8	4.2
Spain (2003)	8.3	12.8	3.9
Italy (2002)	7.1	11.4	3.1
China (1999) Urban[1]	6.7	6.7	6.6
United Kingdom (2002)	6.9	10.8	3.1
Argentina (1996)	6.4	9.9	3.0
Israel (2003)	6.2	10.4	2.1
Brazil (1995)	4.1	6.6	1.8
Mexico (1995)	3.1	5.4	1.0
Greece (2003)	3.4	5.6	1.2
Armenia (2003)	1.8	3.2	0.5
Iran (1991)	0.2	0.3	0.1
Syria (1985)	0.1	0.2	0.0
St Kitts and Nevis (1995)	0.0	0.0	0.0

1 Only selected areas of China have been surveyed.

3.4 **Suicide and age**

Traditionally suicide was considered to increase with age, and that remains the case in many countries. However, in developed countries there has been a significant increase in younger males, where increases of up to three-fold have occurred in the last 30 years, with suicide being one of the three leading causes of death in those under the age of 35. The extent of such changes is sometimes obscured by reductions in elderly suicide tending to compensate for the increase in the young, with a relative constancy of overall suicide rates.

3.5 **Methods of suicide**

There are marked differences in the methods of suicide among countries. The most common methods in England and Wales are hanging, poisoning with drugs, and carbon monoxide poisoning by motor vehicle; in the United States they are fire-arms, hanging, and poisoning with drugs; in Sweden they are poisoning with drugs, hanging, and fire-arms; in Hungary they are hanging, poisoning with drugs, and jumping from a height; in India they are poisoning with pesticides, hanging, and self-immolation by fire; in China they are hanging, drowning, and poisoning with pesticides; and in Australia and New Zealand they are hanging, carbon-monoxide poisoning from motor vehicles, and poisoning with drugs.

The importance of the influence of the predominant method of suicide on a country's suicide rate was highlighted by the sustained reduction in suicide in the United Kingdom following the introduction of non-toxic North Sea gas in 1958. It is also illustrated in those countries where the predominant mode of suicide is agricultural pesticides, as it is probable that this very lethal method of suicide is at least in part responsible for the high rates in countries such as Sri Lanka and in rural China. This contrasts with the ready availability of low lethality tranquilizers being used in Western countries, with less likelihood of death resulting from impulsive overdoses.

3.6 **Variability of suicide rates**

The considerable variation of suicide rates over relatively short periods of time, such as the three-fold increase in suicide in young males in developed countries in the latter decades of the 20th century, has defied simple explanation. Clearly the incidence of mental disorders could not change markedly, and it is challenging to delineate individual psycho-social factors which could be involved. Increasing use of substances, particularly alcohol and amphetamines; changed sex roles; limited employment opportunities; changes in early parenting practices; and changes in the delivery of health care could all be implicated. On the other hand, in the last ten years there have been reductions in suicide in some countries such as the United States, Australia and New Zealand. Again there is no widely accepted simple explanation, although the increased use of antidepressants, as well as broad national suicide prevention initiatives, have probably contributed.

3.7 Attempted suicide

Ten to 20 times the number of those who die by suicide attempt suicide, and estimates in a number of different countries of lifetime risk of a suicide attempt vary between 0.4 and 4.2% of the population. However, these figures are unreliable as many do not come to professional attention.

Young females predominate, particularly in developed countries where less lethal means of suicide are used. The ratio of attempted suicide to suicide also varies depending on the lethality of the most commonly used method. For example, fewer of those who ingest lethal pesticides survive, and therefore the ratio of attempted suicide to suicide is less. That is also the case for attempted suicide in the elderly, where more lethal means are used.

Suicide and attempted suicide are considered to be separate but overlapping populations. However, their antecedents are the same; it is often chance that determines survival or death; and those who attempt suicide are 40 times more likely to die by suicide than a person who has not attempted suicide.

3.8 Suicidal ideation

Suicidal ideation can vary between fleeting thoughts that life is not worth living, to profound delusional beliefs that suicide is the only answer. This variation is reflected in widely differing estimates. Nevertheless, a number of general population studies using different definitions have given a credible figure of about 3 or 4% of the population having a significant degree of suicidal ideation in any one year. Again there is overlap between suicidal ideation and other suicidal behaviours, as follow-up studies have shown a strong association with future attempted suicide and suicide. That is not unexpected, as those who have suicidal ideation have similar developmental and socio-demographic characteristics to those who attempt and die by suicide.

3.9 Self-harm

This usually involves cutting or burning, but can include other self-injurious behaviour. It has also been reported that in a non-treatment sample the commonest form was self-scratching. As many as 15% of adolescents report some degree of self-harm, and much higher rates are reported in adolescent psychiatric patients. The figure reduces to about 4% of the adult population.

It appears to be more a phenomenon of developed countries, and the prevalence has increased markedly in the last three decades. Males and females are equally affected, but females tend to cut, whereas males burn themselves.

Those who self-harm deny suicidal ideation, often citing that it provides a sense of affirmation of the self and relief from feeling nothing. However, they have a greater prevalence of mental disorders, and they also share many of the socio-demographic antecedents of other suicidal behaviours.

3.10 The tipping point and cohort effect

The concept of the 'Tipping Point', which implies that there is a background base rate of a phenomenon resulting from many factors, which when breached for reasons which may not be immediately apparent results in a dramatic increase in that phenomenon, may assist in conceptualizing changes such as the recent increase in self-harm. It also offers some explanation for the observation of a cohort effect, where persons in specific age groups, and who have presumably been exposed to similar broad early life experiences and developmental sociological variables, tend to carry their particular propensity to die by suicide with them throughout life. This cohort effect has been demonstrated in several different countries, and a recent example is the observation that in Australia in the mid 1990s the peak suicide rate was in the 20 to 30-year-old group, and a decade later the peak rate had moved with that cohort, to the 30 to 40-year-old group.

3.11 Limitations of epidemiology in clinical practice

Epidemiological studies provide powerful evidence for the importance of broad psychosocial influences on suicide rates, and they can guide policy makers in regard to broad psycho-social suicide prevention initiatives. However, clinicians must be aware of the ecological fallacy of extrapolating from large epidemiological data sets to an individual person, and when confronted with suicidal patients a more focussed approach is needed.

References

Bertolote, J., Fleischmann, A., De Leo, D. et al. (2005). Suicide attempts, plans, and ideation in culturally diverse sites: the WHO SUPRE-MISS community survey. *Psychol. Med.*, **35**, 1457–65.

Bridge, J.A., Iyengar, S., Salary, C.B. et al. (2007). Clinical response and risk for reported suicidal ideation and suicide attempts in pediatric antidepressant treatment. *J.A.M.A.*, **297**, 1683–96.

Brugha, T., Walsh, D. (1978). Suicide past and present—The temporal constancy of under-reporting. *Br. J. Psychiat.*, **132**, 177–9.

Draper, B.M. (1995). Prevention of suicide in old age. *Med. J. Aust.*, **162**, 533–4.

Goldney, R.D. (1998). Variations in suicide rates: the 'Tipping Point'. *Crisis*, **19**, 136–7.

Grimland, M., Apter, A., Kerkhof, A. (2006). The Phenomenon of Suicide Bombing. *Crisis*, **27**, 107–18.

Hall, W.D., Mant, A., Mitchell, P.B. et al. (2003). Association between antidepressant prescribing and suicide in Australia. *Br. Med. J.*, **326**, 1008–12.

Klonsky, E.D., Muehlenkamp, J.J. (2007). Self-injury: a research review for the practitioner. *J. Clin. Psychol: In Session*, **63**, 1045–56.

Kuo, W.H., Gallo, J.J., Tien, A.Y. (2001). Incidence of suicide ideation and attempts in adults: the 13-year follow-up of a community sample in Baltimore, Maryland. *Psychol. Med.*, **31**, 1181–91.

Morrell, S., Page, A.N., Taylor, R.J. (2007). The decline in Australian young male suicide. *Soc. Sci. Med.*, **64**, 747–54.

Pirkis, J., Burgess, P., Dunt, D. (2000). Suicidal ideation and suicide attempts among Australian adults. *Crisis*, **21**, 16–25.

Sakinovsky, I. (2007). The Current Evidence Base for the Clinical Care of Suicidal Patients: Strengths and Weaknesses. *Can. J. Psychiat.*, **52** (Suppl 1), 7S–20S.

Snowdon, J., Hunt, G.E., (2002). Age, period and cohort effects on suicide rates in Australia, 1919–1999. *Acta Psychiatr. Scand.*, **105**, 265–70.

Wasserman, D., Varnik, A., Dankowicz, M. (1998). Regional differences in the distribution of suicide in the former Soviet Union during perestroika, 1984–1990. *Acta Psychiatr. Scand.*, **98**, 5–12.

World Health Organisation. (1999). Figures and facts about suicide. World Health Organisation, Geneva.

Wikipedia. List of countries by suicide rate. http://en.wikipedia.org/wiki/List_of_countries_by_suicide_rate, Accessed 24/7/07.

Chapter 4

Contributing factors to suicide

> ### Key points
> - The stress-diathesis model is a useful framework to conceptualize suicidal behaviours
> - Psychological autopsy studies demonstrate that 80–90% of suicides had a diagnosable mental disorder at the time of death
> - Population Attributable Risk analyses highlight the importance of mental disorders
> - The presence of even multiple risk factors is not sufficient to adequately explain suicide.

4.1 The stress-diathesis model

There are many theories about the causes of suicidal behaviour and it is challenging to formulate a cohesive conceptual framework within which to operate. A model with clinical utility is the stress-diathesis model, in which the diathesis of longitudinal factors which either raise or lower the threshold to suicidal behaviour is influenced by proximal stressors or triggers which precipitate that behaviour.

Contributors to the diathesis include inherited and developmental factors, mental disorders, personality traits, the presence or absence of interpersonal support systems, societal attitudes and religious beliefs, alcohol and/or other substance abuse, and physical illnesses. Stressors or triggers include factors which contribute to exacerbations of psychiatric illness or acute intoxication with impulsivity, and there is almost invariably a final loss or rejection of an interpersonal nature. A number of these factors can contribute both to the predisposing diathesis, and to the ultimate stress or trigger to suicide. It is also now recognized that there is a subtle interaction between inherited predisposing or susceptibility factors and the environment.

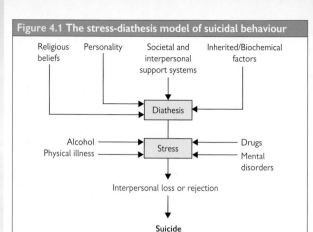

Figure 4.1 The stress-diathesis model of suicidal behaviour

4.2 **The psychological autopsy**

One of the most commonly used research methodologies to delineate contributing factors to suicide is the psychological autopsy, where for almost 50 years data from a variety of clinical and personal biographical sources have been analysed. Studies from no fewer than ten countries have demonstrated consistently that 80–90% of those who died by suicide had mental disorders, particularly depression and substance abuse, at the time of their death. It has also been reported that most of those persons without an axis one diagnosis at the time of death probably had an underlying psychiatric condition that was not detected by the psychological autopsy method.

4.3 **Other research methodologies**

Other research techniques have included twin studies which have confirmed the importance of inherited as well as environmental factors; case-control studies of those who attempt suicide, which have emphasized the importance of mood disorders and substance abuse; large retrospective cohort studies which have demonstrated a graded relationship to attempted suicide of adverse childhood experiences, including emotional, physical, and sexual abuse, household substance abuse, mental illness, and incarceration, and parental domestic violence, separation, or divorce; and longitudinal cohort analyses which have shown that suicidal behaviour is influenced by an accumulation of factors including family history of suicide, childhood sexual abuse, personality factors, peer affiliations and school success or failure.

Danish register research has demonstrated an increasing gradation of suicide risk for those who had mild, moderate or severe depression, confirming clinical beliefs about the prognosis and suicide risk of those with increasing degrees of depression. They have also shown lower risk of suicide for twins, whether the data were examined by cohort, sex or zygosity, results which are supportive of theories embracing the importance of close family ties in suicide prevention.

Other research has also pointed to the importance of the recognition and adequate treatment of mental disorders in suicide prevention. The lack of congruence between the use of psychotropic medication at the time of suicide and the patterns of diagnoses made at psychological autopsy has been noted; there is often a lack of continuity of care; there is frequently an absence of enquiry about suicidal thoughts, particularly in the elderly; and there is often a reduction in the intensity of care prior to suicide.

4.4 Lack of specificity for suicide

It is evident that many of these risk factors, particularly those in childhood and adolescence, are not specific for suicidal behaviours, as they are related to mental disorders in general. Furthermore, it is not necessary to invoke the risk of future suicide as a reason for addressing them. Such issues, for example childhood sexual abuse, parental domestic violence, unemployment, and inadequacies in health services are important in their own right, and they demand the attention not only of health professionals, but also of the community as a whole. It is also important to appreciate that not all risk factors warrant equal attention.

4.5 Relative importance of contributing factors

4.5.1 Population attributable risk studies

Clinicians cannot influence what has happened in the past, although they may wish to lobby for social change that might influence future generations. However, in practical suicide prevention it is important to ensure that a correct perspective be maintained about the relative importance of various risk factors. In this regard Danish register studies have been particularly valuable, as they have used the population attributable risk (PAR) statistic. This is a singularly appropriate statistic for research assessing the differing impact of various contributing factors to suicidal behaviour, as it allows risk factors at the population level to be placed in perspective. The PAR provides a measure of the proportion of a condition that can be associated with exposure to a risk factor, or the proportion of the condition that would be eliminated if the risk factor was not present. It can be illustrated by considering the association between smoking and lung cancer. It is accepted that smoking causes lung cancer, but not in everyone who smokes. The PAR of smoking for lung cancer is about 80%, which means that if all smoking were eliminated, approximately 80% of all lung cancer cases would be eliminated. In an analogous manner, the various PARs for suicidal behaviour can be calculated.

4.5.2 Overwhelming contribution of mental disorders

In a Danish register examination of data for 21,169 suicides and 423,128 comparison subjects, the PAR for suicide of having had a mental disorder necessitating hospital admission was 40.3%, whereas those PARs for other statistically significant contributors, including unemployment, having a sickness-related absence from work, being in the lowest income quartile, and being on a disability or age pension were 2.8%, 6.4%, 8.8%, 3.2% and 10.2%, respectively. While these other issues cannot be ignored, clearly the focus of attention needs to be on those persons who have required hospitalization for mental disorders. Indeed, using the same database and focussing on 496 young suicides between ten and 21 years of age, not only was the presence of a mental disorder the strongest risk factor, but the effect of the parents' socio-economic status decreased after adjusting for family history of mental illness and suicide.

The PAR statistic has been used by other researchers with broadly similar results. For example, there have been a number of studies demonstrating a PAR of approximately 40% of depression for suicide, attempted suicide and even suicidal ideation, and there is an even greater PAR of depression for suicide in the elderly.

Perhaps counter-intuitively, in a study examining the contribution of clinical depression and traumatic and psychosocial events to suicidal ideation, it was found that when multivariate analyses of results were undertaken, which allowed for the interaction of different variables, only clinical depression was significantly associated with suicidal ideation, with a PAR of 47%. Thus no individual traumatic event (e.g. war, life-threatening accident, torture, serious physical attack) or psychosocial event (unplanned loss of job, marriage breakdown, burglary, death of someone close) remained statistically significant. Furthermore, although the lifetime summation of traumatic events attained statistical significance (PAR = 38%), even the summation of psychosocial events did not achieve a statistically significant association with suicidal ideation. This does not mean that those events are not important in themselves; it simply means that they need to be placed in perspective when considering one's management approach for the prevention of suicide.

It is important to appreciate that these PAR results are valid only for the populations studied, that is, in Western countries with well-developed health and social services, and they would not necessarily be applicable to developing countries where there may be alternative public health priorities. For example, countries with high suicide rates due to the ready availability of lethal pesticides would make a greater impact on their suicide rate by addressing the availability of pesticides, rather than by focussing on mental disorders.

4.6 Physical illnesses

Renal haemodialysis and transplantation, neoplasms, particularly those of the head and neck, AIDS/HIV, Systemic Lupus and spinal cord injuries have all been associated with increased rates of suicide.

4.7 Contributing factors are not sufficient to explain suicide

While large scale research has demonstrated conclusively the importance of a number of mental disorders, psycho-social factors and physical illnesses, none of those factors is sufficient to explain suicidal behaviour per se. Indeed, even with an accumulation of such factors, the individual's perception of his or her environment and interpersonal stressors and relationships is still of critical importance in precipitating suicide.

References

Agerbo, E., Nordentoft, M., Mortensen, P.B. (2002). Familial, psychiatric and socioeconomic risk factors for suicide in young people: nested case-control study. *Br. Med. J.*, **325**, 74–78.

Burgess, P., Pirkis, J., Morton. J., Croke, E. (2000). Lessons from a comprehensive clinical audit of users of psychiatric services who committed suicide. *Psychiatr. Serv.*, **51**: 1555–60.

Dube, S.R., Anda, R.F., Felitti, V.J. et al., (2001). Childhood abuse, household dysfunction, and the risk of attempted suicide throughout the life span. Findings from the Adverse Childhood Experiences Study. *J. Am. Med. Assoc.*, **286**, 3089–96.

Ernst, C., Lalovic, A., Lesage, A. et al., (2004). Suicide and no axis I psychopathology. *BMC Psychiat.*, **30**, 4–7.

Fergusson, D.M., Beautrais, A.L., Horwood, L.J. (2003). Vulnerability and resiliency to suicidal behaviours in young people. *Psychol. Med.*, **33**, 61–73.

Goldney, R.D., Dal Grande, E., Fisher, L.J., Wilson, D. (2003). Population attributable risk of major depression for suicidal ideation in a random and representative community sample. *J. Affect. Dis.*, **74**, 267–72.

Hawton, K., Appleby, L., Platt, S., *et al*., (1998). The psychological autopsy approach to studying suicide: a review of methodological issues. *J. Affect. Dis.*, **50**, 269–76.

Hendin, H., Maltsberger, J.T., Haas, A.P., *et al*., (2004). Depression and other affective states in suicidal patients. *Suicide Life Threat. Behav.*, **34**, 386–94.

Isacsson, G., Holmgren, P., Druid, H., Bergman. U. (1999). Psychotropics and suicide prevention. Implications from toxicological screening of 5281 suicides in Sweden 1992–1994. *Br. J. Psychiat.*, **174**, 259–65.

Mann, J.J., Arango, V. (1992). Integration of neurobiology and psychopathology in a unified model of suicidal behavior. *J. Clin. Psychopharmacol.*, **12** (suppl 2), 2S–7S.

Marzuk, P.M., Tardiff, K., Leon, A.C., *et al*., (1995). Use of prescription psychotropic drugs among suicide victims in New York City. *Am. J. Psychiat.*, **152**, 1520–2.

Mortensen, P.B., Agerbo, E., Erikson. T., *et al*. (2000). Psychiatric illness and risk factors for suicide in Denmark. *Lancet*, **355**, 9–12.

National Confidential Inquiry. (2001). Safety first: Five-year report of the National Confidential Inquiry into Suicide and Homicide by People with Mental Illness. Department of Health Publications, London.

Qin. P., Agerbo. E., Mortensen, P.B. (2003). Suicide risk in relation to socioeconomic, demographic, psychiatric, and familial factors: a national register-based study of all suicides in Denmark, 1981–1997. *Am. J. Psychiat.*, **160**, 765–72.

Chapter 5

Mental disorders and the biological substrate of suicide

> **Key points**
>
> - All mental disorders are associated with a higher risk of suicide
> - Mood disorders, schizophrenia and substance abuse are strongly associated with suicide
> - Co-morbidity is common
> - There is an inherited basis to some suicides
> - Serotonin and hypothalamic–pituitary–adrenal axis abnormalities are associated with suicide
> - Biological factors lack specificity for suicide
> - There is an interaction between genetic susceptibility and the environment.

5.1 Mental disorders and suicide

All mental disorders are associated with an elevated risk of suicide. In a meta-analytic review of 44 disorders, 36 had a significantly increased standardized mortality ratio (SMR) for suicide, and five others had a raised SMR that did not attain statistical significance. Only mental retardation and dementia had no increased risk of suicide. Organic mental disorders had the lowest increase in SMR, while mood disorders and schizophrenia had the highest SMRs for suicide.

5.1.1 Mood disorders

A meta-analytic review of 23 follow-up studies of major depression and nine of dysthymia reported that patients with those disorders had a suicide risk of 20 and 12 times respectively that of people with no mood disorder. There is about a 3.5% life time risk of suicide associated with major depression, and psychological autopsy studies have demonstrated that about two-thirds of those who die by suicide have symptoms consistent with major depression at the time of death.

5.1.1.1 *Mood disorders in non-Western countries*

A Taiwanese study used a standardized instrument to assess mood disorders in three different groups, two of aboriginal Taiwanese people and the third of Han Chinese immigrants from mainland China. In each group about 80% of those who died by suicide had symptoms consistent with major depression before their death. This led to the observation that the psychiatric antecedents of suicide were similar in Eastern populations to previous Western studies, and that suicide was of a more universal nature than had previously been assumed, a reference to the prevailing belief that mood disorders were not so prominent in Chinese suicide as had been demonstrated in Western research. These findings have been reinforced by the results of a study of suicides aged 15 to 24 from China, where the importance of the recognition and management of depressive symptoms, as well as restricting access to pesticides was highlighted.

5.1.1.2 *Mood disorders often not diagnosed or treated*

A common theme in these studies is that mood disorders had often not been diagnosed in many of the people who died by suicide, and that even when they had been, those people had often not received adequate treatment for their depressive conditions.

5.1.1.3 *Mood disorders important in young people*

It is sometimes asserted that mood disorders may be of less relevance in suicide in young people. However, a study of 120 suicides under the age of 20 years in New York reported that two-thirds had a mood disorder and 50% had had a duration of symptoms for more than three years, with less than 5% having symptoms for less than three months. This study is particularly important, as it indicates that there is almost invariably a window of opportunity during which the mood disorder could be recognized and treated in young persons.

5.1.1.4 *Mood disorders in attempted suicide*

The association of mood disorders with attempted suicide is sometimes considered less clear-cut. Early studies reported that less than 10% of people who attempted suicide had depressive conditions, but it became apparent that when standardized instruments were used, more depression was delineated than had been the case with clinical reports, with approximately two thirds having a mood disorder. A New Zealand case control study of 'serious' suicide attempts demonstrated that those with a mood disorder were 33 times more likely to have attempted suicide than comparison subjects, and PAR analysis further emphasized the role of depression, particularly in older people, where a PAR of depression for attempted suicide of 73% for those over the age of 55 years indicated that that proportion of serious suicide attempts could be prevented by eliminating depression.

5.1.1.5 *Mood disorders and suicidal ideation*

There is a tendency by some to normalize suicidal ideation as a phase of life or a readily understood reaction to external stressors. While it is probably fair to state that the existential pondering about the meaning of life is part of the human condition, thoughts of actually wishing to die are another matter, although where one draws the line in their delineation will always be open to debate. What can be asserted from a number of studies, using definitions as varied as 'life-weariness' or feeling that life is 'not worth living', is that there are high rates of mental disorders, particularly depression in those endorsing such thoughts, and that the mentally healthy do not have them. There have also been PAR studies which have resulted in similar PARs of depression for suicide, attempted suicide, and suicidal ideation.

5.1.1.6 *Prediction of suicide in mood disorders*

The best predictors of suicide in those with mood disorders are a history of previous suicide attempt, persistent or recurrent depressive symptomatology, particularly if melancholic, and co-morbid alcohol abuse. Factors such as impulsivity and other personality dimensions are less reliable predictors.

5.1.2 **Bipolar disorder**

A meta-analytic review of fourteen reports from seven countries of 3,700 patients found that those with bipolar disorders had a suicide risk 15 times that of those with no disorder. Another study of 12,500 adult private patients recorded a suicide rate of 318 per 100,000 patients per year, and those with bipolar disorders had a seven times greater risk of suicide than those with unipolar depression. In a Finnish study 79% of suicides occurred in the depressed phase, with the most powerful predictors of suicide being a previous suicide attempt and feelings of hopelessness, consistent with other mood disorders.

5.1.3 **Schizophrenia**

Bleuler noted that the most serious of schizophrenic symptoms was the 'suicidal drive', and those with this illness have 30 to 40 times the risk of suicide of the general population, with about a 5% lifetime risk of dying by suicide. Predictors of suicide in schizophrenia include a past history of suicide attempt; co-morbid mood disorders and substance abuse; multiple admissions during the previous year; distressing persistent symptoms; a fear of deterioration with hopelessness and loss of faith in treatment; and concern about side effects of medication. Social isolation and interpersonal rejection are also often observed prior to suicidal behaviour.

5.1.4 **The role of alcohol**

About 40% of those with alcohol dependence will attempt suicide, and up to 7% will die by suicide. Psychological autopsy studies have reported that about 15% of woman and 30% of men who have died by suicide had potentially diagnosable alcohol dependence.

Suicide risk is associated with the availability of alcohol. A comparison of those American states with the minimum legal drinking age of 18 compared to 21 years demonstrated an 8% higher suicide rate in those states with lower legal drinking age, and a Soviet anti-alcohol campaign in Estonia was associated with a reduction in suicide and in blood-alcohol consumption at the time of suicide.

Risk is increased for those with co-morbid major depression and a previous suicide attempt, and other general risk factors include interpersonal rejection, social isolation, co-morbid other substance abuse (particularly cocaine), and a family history of alcohol dependence. Again the risk factors lack specificity, and all those with alcohol dependence should be considered at risk of suicidal behaviour.

5.1.5 Other substances

The contribution of other substances to suicide has been reviewed in a meta-analysis of outcome studies which included alcohol abuse, thereby allowing a comparison. The estimated risks of suicide for alcohol use disorder, opioid use disorder, intravenous drug use, and mixed drug use were ten, 14, 14 and 17 times respectively that of a non-user. It was noted that there were limited data regarding cocaine and cannabis.

Using a differing research methodology, it has been shown that most of the modest increased risk in the association of cannabis and serious suicide attempts in a New Zealand sample was related to confounding factors such as social disadvantage, and that cannabis use was co-morbid with mental disorders which themselves were independently associated with suicidal behaviour. Similarly, in a French study cannabis was not associated with life threatening drug overdoses, whereas that was the case for LSD, buprenorphine and opiates.

5.1.6 Personality disorder

Those with personality disorders, particularly when co-morbid with mood disorders, have an increased risk of suicide. In fact, the diagnostic criteria for the borderline personality disorder include recurrent suicidal behaviour, gestures or threats, or self-mutilating behaviour. These personality disorders are associated with a range of early adverse life experiences.

5.1.7 Co-morbidity

It is increasingly recognized that co-morbidity is important. In a psychological autopsy study of 229 Finnish suicides, the most prevalent axis I diagnoses were depressive disorders (59%), but 43% had alcohol dependence or abuse; 31% had an axis II or personality diagnosis; and 46% had at least one axis III (physical illness) diagnosis. Similar findings have been reported for those who have attempted suicide, and for those with suicidal ideation. In a New Zealand study 57% of people who had made serious suicide attempts had had two or more disorders. Furthermore, although the odds ratio for people with a mood disorder to make a serious suicide attempt was 33 compared with people with no mental disorder, when subjects had had two or more disorders, the odds of a serious suicide attempt increased to 89 times the odds of those with no disorder. Similar findings of comorbidity were found in adolescent suicides in an American study, where mood disorders with conduct disorders and/or substance abuse were common.

5.2 The biological substrate

Bearing in mind the strong association of mental disorders with suicide, and the increasing focus on the biological substrate of psychiatric illness, it is not unexpected that there has been research interest in there being at least some biological contribution to suicidal behaviours.

5.2.1 Inherited factors

There had been clinical observations of an inherited tendency to suicide as long ago as 1790 by Moore, but it was not until the 1970s that the hereditary contribution to suicidal behaviour was given a firm scientific basis when a Danish adoption study examined individuals who were separated at birth from their biological relatives. Using a matched control design, more of the biological relatives of the adopted suicides died by suicide compared to the biological relatives of adopted controls. Consistent with that early study, a recent review of 399 suicide twin pairs demonstrated a 13.2% concordance for suicide in the 129 identical (monozygous) twins, compared to 0.7% concordance for suicide in the 270 non-identical (dizygous) twin pairs. In another study of 5,995 twins, a logistic regression analysis, which controlled for sociodemographic, personality, psychiatric, traumatic event, and family history variables, demonstrated that no less than 45% of the variance in suicidal thoughts and behaviour was related to genetic factors.

5.2.2 Biochemistry of suicide

5.2.2.1 Serotonin

A lowered level of five hydroxy indole acetic acid (5-HIAA) has been found in the cerebrospinal fluid (CSF) of suicide attempters who had used violent methods, and this suggested that it may be a biochemical suicide predictor. This was important, as CSF 5-HIAA is a breakdown product of serotonin, one of the neurotransmitters associated with mood and behaviour disturbances. This finding has been replicated in different centres, and those people who have attempted suicide, particularly by violent means, and who have a low CSF 5-HIAA, have a greater likelihood of subsequently dying by suicide.

The importance of serotonin transmission has also been demonstrated by post-mortem studies, with there being reduced binding to serotonin transporter sites in the ventral prefrontal cortex of the brain of those who died by suicide compared to those who died from other causes. The association between suicidal behaviour and the serotonin system is obviously complex, and it may be related to impulsivity, rather than to any specific psychiatric disorder or suicide per se.

5.2.2.2 *Hypothalamic-pituitary-adrenal axis*

Evidence of the importance of neuro-transmitters and the hypothalamic-pituitary-adrenal axis has emerged from a 15 year follow-up study of depressed patients who had had the dexamethasone suppression test (DST) during their initial assessment. 32 of 78 patients had been non-suppressors, a biological indicator of their depressive condition, and seven of the eight suicides were in that group. None of the demographic and other conventional risk factors distinguished those who died by suicide, but survival analyses demonstrated an estimated risk of suicide in the non-suppressors of 26.8%, compared to only 2.9% for those with a normal DST.

A review of low CSF 5-HIAA and non-suppression on the DST has concluded that they are the most promising biological predictors of suicide, with there being about a 4.5 fold increased risk for each.

5.2.3 Neuropsychological deficits

Recent studies have demonstrated neuropsychological deficits in those with borderline personality disorder and suicidal behaviour, with decision making, visual memory impairment and verbal fluency deficits linked to brain dorsolateral prefrontal and orbitofrontal regions.

5.2.4 Lack of specificity and gene-environment interaction

It is important to note that these biological and inherited predictors lack specificity in the individual person. Furthermore, they do not operate independently, and they do not inevitably lead to suicide in any individual, even if there is a strong family history of suicide. Rather, they can only increase the susceptibility of some individuals to react more severely to stress. This has been shown in research which has demonstrated that persons with one or two copies of the short allele of the serotonin T promoter polymorphism experienced more depression and suicidality in response to stressful life events than those who were homozygous for the long allele. While this has not yet been shown to have direct applicability to suicide per se, it would be unexpected if there was no relationship.

The presence of significant biological and inherited determinants of suicidal behaviour does not negate the importance of the experience of the individual and his or her psychosocial environment. However, there is a need to recognize that mental disorders and biological factors are important, and an appreciation of their role needs to be integrated into potential suicide prevention programmes.

References

Beautrais, A.L., Joyce, P.R., Mulder, R.T. (1999). Cannabis abuse and serious suicide attempts. *Addiction*, **94**, 1155–64.

Beautrais, A.L. (2002). A case control study of suicide and attempted suicide in older adults. *Suicide Life Threat. Behavior.*, **32**, 1–9.

Birckmayer, J., Hemenway, D. (1999). Minimum-age drinking laws and youth suicide, 1970–1990. *Am. J. Public Health*, **89**, 1365–8.

Black, D.W., Monahan, P.O., Winokur, G. (2002). The relationship between DST results and suicidal behavior. *Annals Clin. Psychiat.*, **14**, 83–8.

Caspi, A., Sugden, K., Moffitt, T.E. *et al.* (2003). Influence of life stress on depression: moderation by a polymorphism in the 5-HTT gene. *Science*, **301**, 386–9.

Cheng, A.T. (1995). Mental illness and suicide. A case-control study in east Taiwan. *Arch. Gen. Psychiat.*, **52**, 594–603.

Goldney,R.D., Adam,K.S., O'Brien,J.C., *et al.* (1981). Depression in young women who have attempted suicide: an international replication study. *J. Affect. Disord.* **3**, 327–37.

Harris, E.C., Barraclough, B. (1997). Suicide as an outcome for mental disorders: A meta-analysis. *Br. J. Psychiat.*, **170**, 205–28.

Henriksson, M.M., Aro, H., Marttunen, M.J., *et al.* (1993). Mental disorders and comorbidity in suicide. *Am. J. Psychiat.*, **150**, 935–40.

Kendler, K.S., Kuhn, J.W., Vittum, J., *et al.* (2005). The interaction of stressful life events and a serotonin transporter polymorphism in the prediction of episodes of major depression: a replication. *Arch. Gen. Psychiat.*, **62**: 529–535.

Krysinska, K., Heller, T.S., De Leo, D. (2006). Suicide and deliberate self-harm in personality disorders. *Curr. Opinion Psychiat.*, **19**, 95–101.

LeGris, J., van Reekum, R. (2006). The neuropsychological correlates of borderline personality disorder and suicidal behaviour. *Can. J. Psychiat.*, **51**, 131–42.

Li, X.Y., Phillips, M.R., Zhang, Y.P., *et al.* (2007). Risk factors for suicide in China's youth: a case-control study. *Psychol. Med.* Sept 10, 1 1–10 (Epub ahead of print).

Mann, J.J., Currier, D. (2007). A review of prospective studies of biologic predictors of suicidal behaviour in mood disorders. *Arch. Suicide Res.*, **11**, 3–16.

Palmer, B.A., Pankratz, V.S, Bostwick, J.M. (2005). The lifetime risk of suicide in schizophrenia: a re-examination. *Arch. Gen. Psychiat.*, **62**, 247–53.

Pompili, M., Amador, X.F., Girardi, P., *et al.* (2007). Suicide risk in schizophrenia: learning from the past to change the future. *Ann. Gen. Psychiat.*, **6**: 10 doi: 10.1186/1744–859X-6–10.

Roy, A., Nielsen, D., Rylander, G., Sarchiapone, M. (2000). The genetics of suicidal behaviour. In K. Hawton, K. van Heeringen, eds. *The International Handbook of Suicide and Attempted Suicide*, pp. 209–221, John Wiley & Sons Ltd, Chichester.

Schulsinger, F., Kety, S.S., Rosenthal, D., Wender, P.H. (1979). A family study of suicide. In Schou, M., Stromgren, E., eds. Origin, Prevention and Treatment of Affective Disorders. New York, Academic Press.

Sher, L. (2006). Risk and protective factors for suicide in patients with alcoholism. *Scientific World J.*, **6**, 1405–11.

Shaffer, D., Gould, M.S., Fisher, P., *et al.* (1996). Psychiatric diagnosis in child and adolescent suicide. *Arch. Gen. Psychiat.*, **53**, 339–48.

Statham, D.J., Heath, A.C., Madden, P.A.F., *et al.* (1998). Suicidal behaviour: An epidemiological and genetic study, *Psychol. Med.*, **28**, 839–55.

Tournier, M., Molimard, M., Abouelfath, A. *et al.* (2005). Prognostic impact of psychoactive substances use during hospitalization for intentional drug overdose. *Acta Psychiatr. Scand.*, **112**, 134–40.

Wilcox, H.C., Conner, K.R., Caine, E.D. (2004). Association of alcohol and drug use disorders and completed suicide: an empirical review of cohort studies. *Drug Alcohol Depend.*, **76**: Suppl: S11–19.

Wilhelm, K., Mitchell, P., Niven, H., *et al.* (2006). Life events, first depression onset and the serotonin transporter gene. *Br. J. Psychiatr.*, **188**, 210–15.

Chapter 6

Psychosocial influences on suicidal behaviour

> **Key points**
>
> - The presumed relative importance of broad psycho-social influences as opposed to individual interpersonal factors and mental disorders has fluctuated over time
> - Diverse developmental factors have been associated with adult suicide
> - Proximal situational factors such as the media and access to means of suicide also contribute to suicidal behaviours
> - There have been many interpersonal-psychological theories contributing to our understanding of suicidal behaviour
> - All of these theories have limitations when applied to the individual suicidal person.

The presumed relative importance of broad psychosocial influences, as opposed to individual interpersonal factors and mental disorders in contributing to suicidal behaviours has fluctuated over time. After centuries of an essentially punitive religious view, early 19th century authors had a surprisingly contemporary view of an amalgamation of factors. However, following that there was an increasing focus on broad sociological issues, which culminated in Durkheim's seminal work which, along with the development of psychoanalytic hypotheses, tended to dominate suicide research until the last few decades.

6.1 Broad psychosocial influences

Mid 19th century authors emphasised the importance of the organization of society and of specific social problems, and the influence of civil status, occupation, and literacy were well recognized. Furthermore, altruistic and egotistical suicides had been described by Savage in 1892, prior to Durkheim's more acknowledged sociological theory, including his description of anomic, egoistic, altruistic and fatalistic suicide.

During the 20th century psycho-social factors were explored extensively, and issues such as socio-economic and civil status, and unemployment, as well as concepts of social organization and social integration were noted to be associated with suicidal behaviour. Indeed, their influence is beyond doubt.

Psycho-social causes of suicide are often seen most starkly in those countries or regions which have high suicide rates, and such an attribution has clear face validity. For example, it was considered that the communist oppression of personal freedom in Eastern European countries contributed to their high rates of suicide, and during the first years of Perestroika there was a reduction of suicide in the Russian Federation. However, in the 1990s suicide rates in those countries increased again and the WHO observed that from the sociopolitical perspective, there were reforms which led to western-oriented changes which caused economic and political problems which were distressing for many. A further example is the recently documented phenomenon of high female suicide rates in rural China, which is considered to be related to unique psycho-social pressures on females in modern Chinese society. It is also fair to note that the ready availability of lethal organophosphate pesticides has probably contributed to the high female suicide rate in China, just as it has in other countries such as Sri Lanka and Western Samoa.

Box 6.1 Societal influences

- Socio-economic pressure
- Single civil status
- Unemployment
- Social isolation
- Oppressive political regimes
- Religious faith.

Less commonly referred to from the psycho-social point of view are the extremely low rates of suicide in some countries. Such rates are almost certainly either a reflection of the inadequacy of documentation or a result of state and/or religious sanctions against the reporting of suicide. Traditionally the example of Roman Catholic Ireland has been utilized to illustrate this, as the historically low rates given for Ireland could not be sustained when careful enquiry about religious influence and coronial practices indicated that the true rate was appreciably greater than had hitherto been reported. More recently very low rates of suicide have been reported from some Islamic countries. For example, in Pakistan there had been no official rates of suicide, but data were gleaned from newspaper reports to provide an estimate. Notwithstanding these reservations about the accuracy of suicide rates which may have been reduced artificially by state imposed religious sanctions, it is generally recognized that a strong faith does protect one from suicide to a certain extent.

6.2 Developmental issues

Various research methods have demonstrated the importance of developmental issues such as adverse childhood experiences of emotional, physical and sexual abuse, parental violence and separation, poor peer affiliations, bullying and educational failure in contributing to the propensity to suicidal behaviour in subsequent years. However, the risk factors are broad and lack specificity, being related to the development of mental disorders in general.

Box 6.2 Developmental issues

- Parental violence, separation
- Child abuse, particularly sexual
- Poor peer affiliations
- Bullying
- Educational failure.

The availability of large population data bases has allowed examination of other possible contributing factors. For example, in studies of Swedish males low intelligence at the age of 18 was associated with an increased risk of suicide of two to three times in those with the lowest compared to the highest intelligence test scores; there was an inverse relationship between body mass index (BMI), with suicide decreasing 15% with each five kgm/m^2 increase in BMI; and there was also an inverse relationship between height and suicide risk, with a five cm increase in height being associated with a 9% decrease in suicide. These findings are intriguing, and limited intelligence could be related to an individual's difficulty in problem solving. However, the weight loss did not appear to be related to mental disorders, and, while the inverse association with height could be related to early developmental factors or stigma encountered by short men, these findings defy any simple causal explanation.

37

6.3 More proximal situational factors

At the individual patient level the most important proximal situational factor is almost invariably some form of actual or perceived rejection by another person. However, at the broader community level there are other factors which have the capacity to influence suicidal behaviour.

6.3.1 Access to means of suicide

Access to the means of suicide is influenced by issues such as the presence of natural gas as opposed to coal gas, the availability of firearms, being in a rural environment with pesticides, and being in proximity to railways and jumping sites. Sometimes jumping sites, such as the Golden Gate Bridge, assume folk-lore status in attracting those who are suicidal.

It is increasingly recognized that although some suicidal persons may seek alternative means of suicide if an initial preferred method is eliminated, there is usually an overall sustained reduction in suicide rates following legislation to reduce access to specific means of suicide. In fact, this legislative public health approach has probably had the greatest influence on suicide rates world wide.

6.3.2 **Imitative suicide**

The potential influence of publicity about suicide has been noted for over 200 years. Concern about imitative suicide led to the banning of Goethe's novel *The Sorrows of Young Werther* in some European countries in the 18th century, and in 1841 William Farr stated that 'no fact is better established in science than that suicide (and murder may perhaps be added) is often committed from imitation'. Notwithstanding the strength of that assertion, it took over 100 years before the association was demonstrated statistically. In the last 40 years rigorous research has demonstrated unequivocally that there is an association between publicity about suicide and subsequent increases in suicidal acts.

One study from Germany followed the presentation of a TV series which depicted the death by railway suicide of a 19-year-old male. Against advice this was repeated, thereby allowing a naturalistic A-B-A-B-A research design. Following both screenings there was an increase in imitative suicide, with the greatest and most enduring increase being in those persons closest in age to the model. Another recent Taiwanese study of depressed persons after the suicide of a celebrity reported that 39% were influenced and 5.5% attempted suicide, with the strongest impact being on those who were most severely depressed or who had recently attempted suicide.

The impact of the media is presumed to be based on social learning theory and identification with respected persons who have seemingly resolved their problems by suicide.

6.4 **Interpersonal Psychological theories**

6.4.1 **Traditional psycho-analytic theories**

Traditional Freudian psycho-analytic theory about suicidal behaviour is that it is a reaction to the loss of an ambivalently regarded loved object, with the mixed aggressive feelings being turned inward, rather than being externalized, so much so that suicide has been referred to as murder in the 180th degree. Other early theories included that of Stekel, who suggested that nobody killed themselves unless they had wished for the death of someone else; Menninger focussed on the wish to die, the wish to kill, and the wish to be killed; and object relations theory posits ego-splitting with the wish to kill the introjected object.

6.4.2 More contemporary psychological theories

A 'pre-suicidal syndrome' has been described, in which a constriction of emotion and intellect leads to a narrowing of the range of options. Suicidal behaviour has also been regarded as a 'cry for help', and in that sense it can be interpreted as adaptive from an ethological perspective. These descriptions are consistent with contemporary cognitive theories, which have focussed on hopelessness and a sense of 'entrapment'. Entrapment is the inability to avoid a noxious environment after a loss or humiliation, and recent research has indicated that such feelings can be re-activated by inducing a depressed mood, with suicidal ideation emerging. This cognitive understanding has the potential for the development of specific interventions.

> **Box 6.3 Individual psychodynamics**
>
> - Loss or threatened loss
> - Internalization of aggression
> - Constriction of emotion and intellect
> - Feelings of entrapment
> - Retribution or retaliation
> - Omnipotent mastery
> - Fantasies of re-union.

6.4.3 Insights from psychotherapy

Insights from the psychotherapeutic treatment of suicidal individuals have provided further understanding. Suicidal behaviour is an intensely personal phenomenon, and the emotional pain associated with it has been referred to as 'psychache'. Each suicidal person has his or her own view of the world, which frequently becomes constricted so that alternatives to suicide, or at the very least to seeking temporary oblivion, appear remote. The final act is often precipitated by loss of an interpersonal relationship, and fantasies of retribution or retaliation may be present, so much so that there is sometimes a sense of omnipotence that suicide is not only the solution to his or her problems, but it is also the ultimate method of making others feel sorry for actual or imagined acts against him or her. Other fantasies may be of reunion with significant others who have died, particularly if their death was by suicide.

A detailed analysis of those who died by suicide and who had had at least six visits of psychotherapy has demonstrated that the precipitating event almost always occurred in the setting of one or more intense affective states in addition to depression, and they included feelings of desperation, abandonment, and humiliation. There were also at least one of three behavioural patterns prior to the suicide, including talking about suicide per se, there was a reduction in social and/or occupational functioning, and there was increasing substance abuse.

6.5 Conclusion

Although often seemingly obvious when viewed in retrospect, all of these influences on suicidal behaviour lack specificity in predicting suicide in any individual person. Therefore there is no substitute for careful assessment and the exercise of clinical judgement when confronted with those who may be suicidal.

References

Hendin, H., Maltsberger, J.T., Szanto, K. (2007). The role of intense affective states in signaling a suicide crisis. *J. Nerv. Ment. Dis.*, **195**, 363–8.

Khan, M.M., Reza, H. (2000). The pattern of suicide in Pakistan. *Crisis*, **21**, 31–5.

Magnusson, P.K., Gunnell, D, Tynelius P, *et al.* (2005). Strong inverse association between height and suicide in a large cohort of Swedish men: evidence of early life origins of suicidal behaviour? *Am. J. Psychiat.*, **162**, 1373–5.

Magnusson, P.K., Rasmussen, F., Lawlor, D.A. *et al.* (2006). Association of body mass index with suicide mortality: a prospective cohort study of more than one million men. *Am. J. Epid.*, **163**, 1–8.

McCarthy. P.D., Walsh. D. (1966). Suicide in Dublin. *Br. Med. J.*, **1**, 1393–6.

Schmidtke, A., Häfner, H. (1998). The Werther effect after television films: new evidence for an old hypothesis. *Psychol. Med.*, **18**, 665–76.

Stack, S. (2000a). Suicide: A 15-year review of the sociological literature. Part I: Cultural and economic factors. *Suicide Life Threat. Behavior*, **30**, 145–62.

Stack, S. (2000b). Suicide: A 15 year review of the sociological literature. Part II: Modernization and social integration perspectives. *Suicide Life Threat. Behavior*, **30**, 163–76.

Stack, S. (2003). Media coverage as a risk factor in suicide. *J. Epid. Community Health*, **57**: 238–240.

Williams, J.M.G., Crane, C., Barnhofer, T., Duggan, D. (2005). Psychology and suicidal behaviour: elaborating the entrapment model. In K. Hawton, ed., Prevention and Treatment of Suicidal Behaviour. Oxford University Press, Oxford, pp 71–90.

Chapter 7

An evidence based management approach

> **Key points**
>
> - The low base rate of suicide imposes constraints on the feasibility of using randomized controlled trials to demonstrate the effectiveness of methods of suicide prevention.
> - Alternative research methodologies can be utilized.
> - An integrated management approach addressing both mental disorders and socio-cultural factors is required, with the relative importance of those approaches depending on the individual and the environment.
> - The Haddon Matrix offers a useful framework within which to operate.

7.1 Limitations of the evidence base

The emergence of rigorous evidence-based practice in the latter part of the 20th century led to serious questions being posed about suicide prevention strategies. This was to the extent that it was stated bluntly that no specific interventions had been documented in randomized controlled trials (RCT) to reduce suicide. That such a comment was correct was substantiated by systematic reviews of the treatment literature, and in the late 1990s it was still thought that there was insufficient evidence on which to make firm recommendations about the most effective forms of treatment for those who were suicidal.

7.1.1 The low base rate of suicide

Such pessimistic conclusions need to be considered from the perspective that suicide, for all its drama and the clarity with which retrospective analyses provide, has a low base rate, with the attendant clinical and research limitations that this imposes, particularly in terms of demonstrating the effectiveness of treatments. This is even putting aside the ethical question of placebo treatment for those who are suicidal.

The low base rate, or low incidence of suicide, along with the large number of false positives that are predicted on the basis of conventional suicide risk factors, mean not only that we do not have reliable predictors of suicide in the individual person, but they impose limitations on the research methodologies which can be utilised to demonstrate the effectiveness of specific treatments. For example, to demonstrate a 15% reduction in suicide in those discharged from psychiatric hospitals, where there is a 0.9% chance of suicide in the subsequent year, over 140,000 patients would be required in the research sample. Similarly, to demonstrate the effectiveness of suicide prevention in other high-risk populations, to reduce the suicide rate in doctors and farmers by 25%, 25,000 and 33,000 subjects respectively would be required for RCTs.

The numbers required to demonstrate the effectiveness of the prevention of repetition of attempted suicide are less than for suicide *per se*, but still considerable. Even combined data from 20 RCTs in a meta-analysis were too few to detect differences in outcome. It has been noted that if the anticipated attempted suicide rate was 10% in a treatment group vs 15% in the control group, with α set at 0.05 and β set at 0.2, 687 subjects would be required in each group. Naturally, multi-centred collaborative trials could be utilized to enhance numbers. However, the logistical demands, let alone the financial requirements, are daunting. For example, in a World Health Organisation/European Union follow-up study at nine centres of 4,163 persons who had attempted suicide, for a variety of reasons only 2,432 subjects were asked to participate in a follow-up study, and of those only 1,145 were re-assessed after one year. This provided what the researchers termed a "gross completion rate" of 28% of the original sample, or a "net completion rate" of 47% of those who agreed to participate. When the need for randomization of treatment and control subjects is added, the challenge in designing outcome research in this area is obvious, even with highly motivated researchers in dedicated centres such as in this study.

7.2 The need for alternative research methodologies

In view of these reports, those charged with responsibility for suicide prevention could be forgiven for being pessimistic. However, the results of such reviews not only fail to support long held clinical beliefs, but they also ignore research methodologies other than RCTs. When a more pragmatic approach is adopted and other research strategies are utilized, there is a considerable body of evidence which can give clinicians confidence in their practice to reduce suicidal behaviour.

As will be evident from considering the diverse contributing factors to suicidal behaviour, there are many areas where intervention can reasonably be addressed. However, not all contributing factors have equal impact; contributing factors vary from country to country and between regions in the same country; and clinicians faced with individual suicidal patients may need to utilize a different approach with differing priorities to those responsible for broader suicide prevention initiatives.

7.2.1 An integrated management approach

This is illustrated by referring to a model which has attempted to reconcile the widely differing suicide rates of individual countries with the presumed impact of socio-cultural factors upon a broadly similar base rate of suicide due to biological factors.

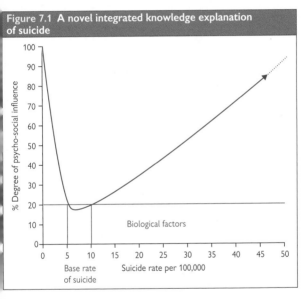

Figure 7.1 A novel integrated knowledge explanation of suicide

This model assumes a base rate of approximately five to ten suicides per 100,000 population, with this range being related to inherited factors, such as serotonin transporter gene anomalies, interacting with a relatively benign socio-cultural environment with good inter-personal and community supports. The focus of management in such situations should be on the optimum treatment of mental disorders, albeit with an awareness of the contribution of psycho-social stressors to even the most biological of mental disorders.

Figures differing markedly from this range indicate an increasing impact of socio-cultural factors. Extremely low figures lack credibility, and are undoubtedly attributed to socio-political pressures or inadequate data gathering. However, for clinicians working in countries with very high rates of suicide, wider societal issues such as adverse socio-cultural circumstances or the ready availability of a method of suicide, such as pesticides, will be of greater importance in reducing suicide at the community level, although the principle of thorough clinical assessment of the individual suicidal person will always be required. Individual treatment decisions need to be made on the basis of the best available clinical evidence, but at the same time clinicians can lobby health administrators and politicians for broader societal change.

7.2.2 The prevention paradox

Some clinicians and adherents to RCT evidence based management approaches are sceptical about the capacity of broad community initiatives to effect change. Such scepticism should be allayed by the marked changes in suicide rates following legislation to reduce access to means of suicide. However, less dramatic changes are more the norm, and there are formidable obstacles in determining specific causality if and when changes occur. Nevertheless, it must be acknowledged that even small changes in attitudes, perceptions and actions as a result of broad community programmes could reduce suicidal behaviour. This is consistent with the public health perspective of the "prevention paradox", where it has been noted that a virtually imperceptible effect on an individual may in fact result in a measurable change at the population level. This is also consistent with the tipping point explanation for marked changes in the prevalence of suicidal behaviours over relatively short time periods.

7.2.3 The Haddon Matrix

Whilst the previously noted stress/diathesis conceptualization of suicidal behaviour is probably the most accepted in clinical practice, another model which allows a potentially clearer delineation of where evidence based interventions are feasible, and by whom, is the Haddon Matrix. This is a public health model, based on the host or individual person; the agent or means of suicidal behaviour; and the environment, including the person's personal and community relationships.

7.3 A practical approach

Very few of the intervention studies referred to in subsequent chapters meet RCT requirements because of the low base rate of suicide and the impossibility of recruiting sufficient numbers. However, research using a variety of differing methodologies provides persuasive evidence for the effectiveness of a number of specific interventions.

Table 7.1 HADDON Matrix of factors influencing suicidal behaviour and its outcome

	Individual	Means of suicidal	Environment behaviour
Pre-suicidal factors	• Age, • Gender • Personality • Mental disorders • Substance abuse • Inherited factors • Physical illness	Accessibility of— • drugs • firearms • pesticides • jumping sites	• Personal relationships • Community support • Media influences
Suicidal behaviour	• Substance intoxication • Inter-personal rejection • Suicidal intent	Lethality of method	• Proximity to others • Likelihood of discovery/prevention
Post-suicidal factors	• Help seeking • General health • Compliance with treatment	Effectiveness of acute and follow-up treatment	• Availability of treatment • Social and personal support network

References

Bille-Brahe, U., Kerkhof, A., De Leo, D., et al. (1996). A repetition-prediction study on European parasuicide populations. *Crisis*, **17**, 22–31.

Eddleston, M., Buckley, N.A., Gunnell, D., et al. (2006). Identification of strategies to prevent death after pesticide self-poisoning using a Haddon matrix. *Inj. Prev.*, **12**, 333–7.

Goldney, R.D. (2003). A novel integrated knowledge explanation of factors leading to suicide. *New Ideas Psychol.*, **21**, 141–6.

Goldney, R.D., (2005) Suicide prevention : a pragmatic review of recent studies. *Crisis* **26**, 128–40.

Gunnell, D., Frankel, S. (1994). Prevention of suicide: aspirations and evidence. *Br. Med. J.*, **208**, 1227–33.

Hawton, K., Arensman, E., Townsend, E., et al. (1998). Deliberate self-harm: the efficacy of psycho-social and pharmacological treatments. *Br. Med. J.*, **317**, 441–7.

Lewis, G., Hawton, K., Jones, P. (1997). Strategies for preventing suicides. *Br. J. Psychiat.*, **171**, 351–4.

Rose, G. (1992). The Strategy of Preventive Medicine. Oxford, Oxford University Press.

Chapter 8

Initial assessment and management

Key points

- Establish rapport
- Assess suicidal intent
- Enquire about means of suicide
- Assess mental state
- If no mental disorder, offer precautionary follow-up and advise about alternative problem solving methods
- If a mental disorder is present, arrange appropriate management
- Follow-up.

Not all in the helping professions should feel obliged to provide on-going management of those who are suicidal. We all have our preferred areas of expertise, and there may be recognized transference and counter-transference issues which we appreciate would compromise our effectiveness. However, all should have some capacity for conducting the initial assessment and, if indicated, for making recommendations for further management.

The fundamentals of assessing and managing a suicidal person are to establish rapport; to assess suicidal intent; to determine if there is a mental disorder which requires ongoing management, and if so to provide that; and if there is no mental disorder, to offer follow-up support even it if may appear to be rejected.

8.1 Initial contact

8.1.1 Establish rapport

The initial contact with a suicidal person is particularly important, but it often occurs in less than ideal circumstances, such as in the home or in a busy emergency room. There may be concerns about the physical condition of the patient and he or she may be antagonistic towards others, including clinicians, as almost invariably the suicidal behaviour will have been precipitated by perceived rejection by someone significant.

Considerable expertise and patience may be required to establish rapport. This may be achieved by emphasizing that you want to try and understand what has happened to the individual person, and that a certain amount of time has been set aside to listen. Courtesy and respect for the individual is essential, and it is important to provide privacy. It is unrealistic to expect someone to divulge sensitive personal information unless confidentially is assured.

The individual should be given the opportunity to express his or her thoughts and feelings and allowed to discharge pent-up and repressed emotions. This catharsis should put the person's suicidal intentions at least temporarily on hold. It is best to avoid challenging, closed questions such as 'Do/did you really want to die?'. Open-ended enquiry such as 'What are/were your feelings about living and dying?' is far more likely to elicit useful information.

8.1.2 Suicidal intent

Detailed enquiry about the circumstances of the suicidal behaviour is essential in order to make a judgement about the degree of suicidal intent, both from the subjective point of view of the individual and also from the clinician's objective view. Sometimes suicidal intent is denied or minimized, and the circumstances surrounding the suicidal behaviour and the description of significant others need to be considered. The following are important:

- What led up to the suicidal behaviour?
- How much planning has there been?
- Was the behaviour pre-meditated or impulsive?
- What were the person's feelings about living and dying?
- What was the knowledge and expectation of the person about the potential lethality of their actions?
- Have there been any acts in anticipation of death, such as making a will or saying goodbye to others?
- Has suicidal intent been conveyed to others?
- Is the suicidal behaviour aimed at manipulating others in the environment?
- Has the person acted to gain help during or after the attempt?
- Have precautions been taken against discovery or intervention during the attempt?
- Has the behaviour occurred in isolated circumstance, or where others could intervene?

Suicidal intent scales have been devised, and high scores are associated with an increased risk of suicide in the long term. However, they are of limited clinical utility, although their use can ensure that clinicians address fully the individual components of suicidal intent.

8.1.3 Means of suicide

It is important to ask about the availability of means of suicide, and the focus of this enquiry will depend on the predominant method of suicide in the region. The availability of lethal medications or agricultural poisons should be addressed, and if firearms are available, local laws about their possession may need to be invoked in regard to notifying firearms regulatory authorities. Tact is required, and concern for safety rather than punitive action should be emphasized.

8.2 Mental state examination

An integral part of the assessment of suicidal persons is the mental state examination, which is analogous to the physical examination in general clinical practice. This occurs concurrently with the initial assessment of suicidal intent, and involves evaluating the person's appearance and behaviour in the interview, their speech pattern, their affective state, the presence of psychotic phenomena such as hallucinations and delusions, their cognitive state which may have been compromised by their suicidal behaviour, their capacity for introspection and insight, and their ability to form a therapeutic relationship.

Bearing in mind the importance of mood disorders in contributing to suicidal behaviour, it is prudent to ask specific questions about depression. The questions 'during the past month have you often been bothered by feeling down, depressed or hopeless?' and 'during the past month have you often been bothered by little interest or pleasure in doing things?', followed by 'is this something with which you would like help?' have a high degree of sensitivity and specificity for delineating major depression.

8.2.1 Ominous clinical features

There are a number of ominous clinical features that should alert the clinician to a greater likelihood of suicide. The expression of high suicidal intent, with severe depression, agitation, guilt, desperation, abandonment, humiliation, hopelessness, and a constriction of interest or self-absorption, should be taken particularly seriously. So should malignant alienation, a syndrome seen in those who have exhausted the patience and resources of friends and relatives and also of the helping professions, sometimes resulting in them being subjected to disparaging comments from others, including clinicians.

Although these factors are associated with suicide risk, the dilemma is that they still lack specificity for suicide per se, even though clinical experience mandates that they should be acted upon.

8.3 **Hospitalization**

Hospitalization may be necessary because of the physical effects of suicidal behaviour; if there are specific suicide plans, particularly with associated impulsivity; if an active psychotic illness is present; and if there is profound depression, hopelessness, and nihilism. The degree of social support a patient has may also influence the decision to hospitalize.

Compulsory admission using appropriate mental health legislation may be required to reduce the risk to the patient or others. Legislation requires careful interpretation, as it is onerous to treat people against their wishes. However, it can be argued that erring on the side of caution in this clinical situation mandates imposing constraints on a patient in order to buy time for the suicidal impulse to dissipate. In these circumstances it is important to emphasize to the suicidal person and his or her relatives and friends that this is done because of concern for the person, not to punish him or her.

There are no RCTs to either endorse or refute the wisdom of compulsory admission for some of those who have attempted suicide, and it is a clinical decision which sometimes must be made with incomplete information. However, an Australian study found that those who absconded from a general hospital after attempting suicide by drug overdose had a 10.8 times risk of subsequent suicide compared with others who had attempted suicide, whereas those who were transferred compulsorily to a psychiatric hospital had 3.2 times risk of suicide. Naturally one can not draw definitive conclusions from such results, but it is evident that both groups were at high risk of suicide, and it could be argued that those who absconded were denied the potential benefit of compulsory hospitalization. Furthermore, a recent UK case-control study of in-patient suicide found that patients who had been detained for compulsory treatment were less likely to die by suicide.

8.4 **Benefits of comprehensive initial assessment**

The importance of comprehensive initial assessment has been illustrated by studies which have followed up those who were not assessed adequately in emergency departments. One study found that deliberate self-harm patients who left an accident and emergency department without a psychiatric assessment not only had a greater past history of self-harm, but they were more likely to self-harm again in the subsequent year than a matched comparison group who had been assessed. Similar findings from another study showed that patients who had deliberately self-poisoned and who had not received psychosocial assessment were more likely to poison themselves again. Furthermore, those investigators calculated that only twelve patients needed to receive a psychosocial assessment to prevent one repetition of self-poisoning, a result which would have a marked effect on busy emergency departments.

8.5 Need for subsequent management

After the initial assessment, the opportunity to have expressed their thoughts and feelings, with resultant catharsis, may have been sufficient for some suicidal people. However, even if there is no mental disorder and the suicidal thoughts and actions have resulted in positive changes in personal relationships, it is important to emphasize that there are other options besides suicidal behaviour, and follow-up should be offered to reinforce alternative problem solving methods.

If mental disorders are present, standard management practices should be provided, along with clear advice about alternative problem solving methods.

Box 8.1 Fundamentals of management

- Establish rapport
- Assess suicidal intent
- Ensure safety
- Assess mental state
- If no mental disorder:
  - catharsis + follow up
- If interpersonal/family issues:
  - catharsis + problem solving approach
  - consider referral to psychologist or social worker
- If mental disorder:
  - catharsis + standard management for that disorder
  - appropriate psychotherapeutic support
  - consider psychiatric referral and psychotropic medication if indicated.

References

Arroll, B., Goodyear-Smith, F., Kerse, N. *et al.* (2006). Effect of the addition of a 'help' question to two screening questions on specificity for diagnosis of depression in general practice: diagnostic validity study. *Br. Med. J.*, **331**, 884–7.

Beck, A.T., Schuyler, D., Herman, I. (1974). Development of suicidal intent scales. In The Prediction of Suicide, eds. A.T. Beck, H.L.P. Resnik, D.J. Lettieri, The Charles Press, Bowie, Maryland.

Hickey, L., Hawton, K. Fagg, J., Weitzel, H. (2001). Deliberate self-harm patients who leave the accident and emergency department without a psychiatric assessment: a neglected population at risk of suicide. *J. Psychosom. Res.*, **50**, 87–93.

Hunt, I.M., Kapur , N., Webb, R. *et al.* (2007). Suicide in current psychiatric in-patients: a case-control study. The National Confidential Inquiry into Suicide and Homicide. *Psychol. Med.*, **37**, 831–7.

Kapur, N., House, A., Dodgson, K. *et al.* (2002). Effect of general hospital management on repeat episodes of deliberate self poisoning: Cohort study. *Br. Med. J.*, **325**, 866–7.

Reith, D.M., Whyte, I., Carter, G. *et al.* (2004). Risk factors for suicide and other deaths following hospital treated self-poisoning in Australia. *Aust. N.Z. J. Psychiat.*, **38**, 520–5.

Chapter 9

Non-pharmacological approaches

Key points

- All suicidal persons warrant emotional support, the nature and intensity of which depend on the presence and type of mental disorder.
- Dialectical Behaviour Therapy is specifically effective for those with Borderline personality disorder.
- Other treatments include Cognitive Behaviour Therapy, Interpersonal Therapy, Problem Solving Therapy and Mindfulness based Cognitive Therapy.
- The risk of dependence needs to be balanced between encouraging independence and being perceived as rejecting.
- Broader non-pharmacological approaches include crisis centres and volunteer organizations.

9.1 The individual approach

All those who are suicidal warrant some form of emotional support, or psychotherapy in its broadest sense, the nature and intensity of which depend on the presence and type of mental disorder. If no mental disorder has been delineated after full assessment, a follow-up visit should be offered, and if accepted a problem-solving approach can be adopted in order to learn more adaptive ways of coping in the future. If a mental disorder is present, standard treatments should be followed, albeit with a focus on providing alternative coping strategies to suicidal behaviour. If medication is indicated, that does not obviate the need for concurrent emotional support. The nature of this will depend on the age of the patient, and it may involve parents of children and adolescents, or other family members or friends of older patients.

The demonstrated effectiveness of any specific psychotherapeutic intervention only dates from the development of the Dialectical Behaviour Therapy (DBT) model.

9.1.1 **Dialectical Behaviour Therapy (DBT)**

DBT involves cognitive, behavioural, and supportive techniques specifically for those with borderline personality disorder. A number of studies have demonstrated a reduction in the number and severity of suicide attempts, and also a decrease in hospital admissions.

It is fair to state that the DBT model of treatment is demanding on both patient and therapist. It addresses increasing the patient's behavioural capabilities; improving motivation for appropriate behaviour; the structure of the treatment environment to reinforce appropriate behaviour; the generalizability of gains; and also the therapist's capabilities and motivation. It is intensive, with weekly individual psychotherapy for one hour; there is two and a half hours per week of group skills training; telephone consultations are on an as needs basis; and there are weekly therapist team meetings as well.

Variations on this rigorous DBT approach have been effective for borderline patients in other studies, but a recent multi-centre randomized trial utilizing manual assisted Cognitive Behaviour therapy, which incorporated DBT concepts, found no difference in the repetition of deliberate self-harm between the experimental and treatment-as-usual groups. However, subjects were not chosen for their clinical diagnosis, as is the case for DBT.

Despite that negative finding, other studies have demonstrated the effectiveness of Cognitive Behaviour Therapy and Interpersonal Therapy in reducing depression, suicidal ideation and repeated self harm after deliberate self poisoning, and Problem Solving Therapy has resulted in reduced depression and hopelessness in deliberate self-harm patients. More recently Mindfulness-based Cognitive Therapy has shown promise in reducing the likelihood of re-emergence of suicidal ideation in those who have had it in the past. Patients in all of these studies did not have psychotic illnesses, although they would not necessarily preclude such persons from having the potential benefit of these additional psychotherapies.

Box 9.1 Individual psychotherapies

- All suicidal persons should be offered support of some type
- Dialectical Behaviour Therapy is specific for those with Borderline Personality Disorder
- Other psychotherapies include:
  - Cognitive Behaviour Therapy
  - Interpersonal Therapy
  - Problem Solving Therapy
  - Mindfulness Based Cognitive Therapy.

The principles which form the basis of the most common approaches are as follows:

9.1.2 Cognitive Behaviour Therapy (CBT)

The aim of CBT is to identify the patient's errors in cognition of self, to modify these by cognitive and behavioural techniques, and to guide the person towards mastery of their thoughts and actions, thereby minimizing the likelihood of further suicidal behaviour.

CBT is based on the observations that those who are suicidal see themselves as inadequate and unworthy; they view any interaction with others as extremely demanding and tend to minimize any successful experiences; and they tend to view the future with negative expectancies, anticipating that any initiatives are doomed from the start. Therapy is designed to counteract these errors of cognition, and involves both cognitive and behavioural techniques.

Patients are asked to define specific thoughts which may be plausible to them, but which can in fact be readily seen to be idiosyncratic and self-defeating. The therapist then assists the patient in what is in essence a scientific examination of the statement. This is done in a non-judgemental manner, the patent inaccuracy of the thought is pointed out, and the patient is invited to generate alternative hypotheses to explain their thinking. This is an important aspect of identifying maladaptive assumptions, as it provides the patient with alternative modes of thinking that are less self-deprecating.

To illustrate the point, suicidal patients frequently believe they are failures in all aspects of their lives. By asking them to step outside themselves and view themselves as others would, areas of competence such as the ability to work, play sport or to have raised children can invariably be elicited, and the original assumption can be seen to be false. The therapist can then ask how it is that these successes have occurred, thus manoeuvring patients into acknowledging that they must have had some good points to have contributed to that successful outcome.

The behavioural component of CBT is similar in principle and is based on scheduling activities that can actually be mastered by the patient, and which provide alternatives to suicidal behaviour. Goals which are said to be impossible are identified and then broken down into graded tasks, and the successful completion of each task provides immediate confirmation that a patient is competent. Such activities can be done in imagination as a form of 'cognitive rehearsal' or as role playing, but it is essential that real life tasks be done promptly, thereby providing gratification and reassurance of the patient's mastery.

An important aspect of CBT is to have an agenda for each session with a list of priorities which can be achieved. It is also helpful to give 'homework', where maladaptive thoughts are recorded along with alternative hypotheses. Scheduled activities should be noted in order to monitor the outcome of the graded steps towards achieving the goals of treatment. Some patients may require focus upon much smaller steps than others, and it is important that continual feedback of achievements be given at each session.

It is essential to maintain a problem-oriented stance and keep patients focused on concrete achievable goals, as by this method a person's self-esteem may be repeatedly reinforced and suicidal behaviour is less likely.

9.1.3 Interpersonal Therapy (IPT)

The overall aim in IPT is to elicit, clarify and place into perspective those feelings that have arisen from interaction with others, and which have led to suicidal ideation or behaviour.

It is based on the premise that suicidal behaviour occurs in a psychosocial and interpersonal context. The emphasis is on current problems, anxieties and frustrations, with an effort being made to define problems in 'here and now' terms. Loss and threatened loss are crucial, as are ambivalent feelings about them. Eliciting mixed feelings about loss is particularly important, as one of the classic formulations of suicidal behaviour is that the suicidal person is unable to come to terms with angry feelings regarding losses, for fear of guilt about those emotions. Instead, these angry feelings are turned inwards against the self, thereby precipitating the suicidal behaviour. The therapist must be aware of such feelings and encourage their expression.

Sometimes losses may not be readily apparent, and in patients in whom denial is prominent, a careful history elucidating relationships with parents, siblings, children and significant others is necessary. It is important to remember that suicidal behaviour has a large interpersonal/communication component, and it almost invariably occurs in the context of interpersonal rejection. By exploring and clarifying feelings associated with that, reported suicidal behaviour is less likely to occur.

9.1.4 Problem Solving Therapy

This is based on the premise that symptoms are related to everyday problems, which if solved the symptoms will be alleviated. Initially the patient describes their symptoms and problems, and they are linked, thereby giving a rationale for addressing the problem. Major problems can be dissected into their components, and potential solutions can be generated by the patient and therapist, and the preferred solution can be determined by logical analysis. The solution can then be practised in imagination, and role playing can also be utilized. Then the individual is encouraged to use the new problem solving techniques in their everyday life and personal relationships.

Review of progress is essential, as is encouragement to persist, albeit sometimes with modification of the preferred problem solving technique.

9.1.5 Mindfulness Based Cognitive Therapy (MBCT)

MBCT uses aspects of Cognitive Therapy with meditation techniques from Buddhism. It is intensive and requires considerable commitment. There are seven weekly two hour classes, and an all day practice between the sixth and seventh classes, as well as individual daily practice. Various aspects of bodily sensations are focussed on, to the extent that participants are aware of small experiences that previously might have passed unnoticed. The role of negative thoughts and ruminations in perpetuating distress is addressed, but more in the sense of acceptance that they are simply thoughts and not necessarily reflections of reality. While this approach shows promise, it is important to note that it is not an acute treatment, but a technique to prevent relapse.

9.2 The risk of dependence

Therapists must be willing to listen to the demands of suicidal patients, but these demands can not be met unconditionally, and the focus must be on the person accepting responsibility for his or her own actions. There is a fine line between fostering independence and appearing to reject those who are suicidal. The fostering of independence can be aided by the therapist making it clear to the patient that his or her involvement will be time-limited and then, at the end of that time, expressing confidence in the person's ability to cope in a more adaptive manner when future crises arise, even though the person may not be completely at ease with himself or herself.

While this approach is appropriate for most suicidal patients, some, such as young adults with few family and social supports, those with borderline personalities, and patients with chronic psychiatric illness, may require longer term contact, with encouragement to manage their condition on a long term basis with appropriate professional support and back-up for crises.

9.3 Broader non-pharmacological approaches

9.3.1 Crisis centres and the role of volunteers

The first telephone crisis centres to prevent suicide were established in the United States in the early 20th century. However, the main impetus to their development was provided by Chad Varah, a clergyman, who founded the Samaritans in England in 1953. Since then there have been Crisis centres in many countries, usually under the auspices of volunteer organizations such as the Samaritans, Befrienders International, the International Federation of Telephonic Emergency Services (IFOTES), and Lifeline. Formidable methodological problems exist in demonstrating their effectiveness, but a review of 14 studies concluded that overall there was an impact on suicidal behaviour in those areas which had such centres. Furthermore, recent studies have found significant decreases in measures of suicidality between the beginning and end of telephone counselling sessions.

The principles behind Crisis centres are that they are readily accessible by phone; they are available 24 hours a day; they are acceptable to some who may not access alternative services; and some prefer their anonymity. Non-judgemental acceptance of tele phone calls is extended to face-to-face contact in some volunteer organizations, where the principles of befriending apply. This may involve regular contact up to once a week, talking, listening and "being there" for practical issues.

The effectiveness of befriending has been demonstrated in reducing symptoms of chronic depression in women in London. It was also applied in a project from Sri Lanka, initiated by Sumithrayo, a volunteer organization dedicated to suicide prevention. In response to suicidal behaviour in rural areas, befriending support was offered to a village with another village used as a comparison. The village with the intervention had had 13 suicides and 18 other episodes of self harm in the six years before the programme, but there were no examples of suicidal behaviour in the subsequent four and a half years. That contrasted with the comparison village which had previously had 16 suicides and 25 other episodes of self harm, and which had a further three suicides and ten other episodes of self harm in the next two years, following which the investigators extended the programme to that village.

9.3.2 Innovative approaches
9.3.2.1 *Post cards*
A deceptively simple form of ongoing contact with suicide attempters in the United States resulted in a significant reduction in suicide for the duration of the contact. Those who had attempted suicide were contacted one month after their suicide attempt and those who had not pursued further treatment were randomly assigned to contact and no contact groups. The contact group received correspondence each month for four months, then every two months for eight months and then every three months for a further four years, a total of five years and 24 contacts per person. The contact usually involved a short letter, but sometimes a phone call, and each letter was worded slightly differently and included responses if previous contact had been reciprocated. The letters simply noted that it was some time since the person had been at the hospital, that it was hoped all was well, and that they could make contact if they wished.

Over a five-year period there was a statistically significant decrease in death by suicide for those who had had contact when compared to the no contact group. However, longer-term follow-up indicated that the difference became insignificant, and the suicide rates were identical after 14 years. Nevertheless, the data demonstrated a significant difference in the first five years, and it is reasonable to suggest that if further contact had been continued beyond that time, more encouraging long-term results might have eventuated.

A recent replication study in Australia with a two year follow-up found that although the number of individuals who repeated self-poisoning was not reduced, there was a statistically significant halving of the overall repetition of self-poisoning.

3.2.2 *Tele-check and Tele-help*

A study of elderly persons discharged from hospital in Italy involved regular check of patients by telephone, on average twice a week, and patients also had a Tele-Help component of a portable device which allowed them to send an alarm signal if they needed help. Over a ten year period there were only six suicides compared to an expected 21 for that population of 18,641 elderly persons, a statistically significant difference.

These innovative low-cost interventions warrant further replication in different settings to confirm their effectiveness.

9.4 Common therapeutic components

There are commonalities in these non-pharmacological approaches. Suicidal persons are assessed and treated with respect and seriousness; the individual face-to-face interventions are not open-ended, but structured with agreed objectives and they may utilise a manual-based approach; the Crisis centres and volunteers provide a readily accessible and non-judgemental point of contact which can buy time to allow the suicidal crisis to dissipate; and the innovative techniques embody a sense of reaching out and offering support. These overall approaches embrace the concepts of warmth, genuineness and accurate empathy, which have been shown to be of benefit in effective psychotherapy. They are also consistent with what has been described as enhancing a sense of 'connectedness to others'.

Box 9.2 Common therapeutic components

- A respectful serious approach
- Non-judgemental
- Embody warmth, genuineness and empathy
- Provide a sense of 'connectedness to others'.

References

Berk, M.S., Henriques, G.R., Warman, D.M. *et al.* (2004). A cognitive therapy intervention for suicide attempters: an overview of the treatment and case examples. *Cog. Behav. Practice*, **11**, 265–77.

De Leo, D., Marirosa, D.B., Dwyer, J. (2002). Suicide among the elderly: the long-term impact of a telephone support and assessment intervention in northern Italy. *Br. J. Psychiat.*, **181**, 226–9.

Carter, G.L., Clover,K., Whyte, I.M. *et al.* (2007). Postcards from the EDge: 24-month outcomes of a randomised controlled trial for hospital treated self-poisoning. *Br. J. Psychiatr.*, **191**, 548–53.

Frank, J. (1971). Therapeutic factors in psychotherapy. *Am. J. Psychother.* **15**, 350–61.

Gould, M.S., Kalafat, J., Harrismunfakh, J.L., Kleinman, M. (2007). An evaluation of crisis hotline outcomes. Part 2: Suicidal callers. *Suicide Life Threat. Behav.*, **37**, 338–52.

Lester, D. (1997). The effectiveness of suicide prevention centers: a review. *Suicide Life Threat. Behav.*, **27**, 304–310.

Linehan, M.M., Comtois, K.A., Murray, A.M. *et al.* (2006). Two-year Randomized Controlled Trial of follow-up of Dialectical Behavior Therapy vs therapy by experts for suicidal behaviors and borderline personality disorder. *Arch. Gen. Psychiat.*, **63**: 757–66.

Maracek, J., Ratnayeke, L. (2001). Suicide in rural Sri Lanka: assessing a prevention programme. In O.T. Grad, ed., Suicide Risk and Protective Factors in the new Millenium. Ljubljana, Cankarjev dom, pp. 215–219.

McMain, S. (2007). Effectiveness of psychosocial treatments on suicidality in personality disorders. *Can. J. Psychiat.*, **52** (Suppl 1): 1035–45.

Motto, J.A., Bostrom, A.G. (2001). A randomized controlled trial of post-crisis suicide prevention. *Psychiat. Serv.*, **52**, 828–33.

Mynors-Wallis, L. (2001). Problem-solving treatment in general psychiatric practice. *Adv. Psychiat. Treat.*, **7**, 417–25.

Scott, V. (1996). Reaching the suicidal: the volunteer's role in preventing suicide. *Crisis*, **17**, 102–4.

Tyrer, P., Thompson, S., Schmidt, U. *et al.* (2003). Randomised controlled trial of brief cognitive behavior therapy versus treatment as usual in recurrent deliberate self-harm: the POP-MACT Study. *Psychol. Med.* **33**, 969–76.

Williams, J.M.G., Duggan, D.S., Crane, C., Fennel, M.J.V. (2006). Mindfulness-based cognitive therapy for prevention of recurrence of suicidal behavior. *J. Clin. Psychol.*, **62**, 201–10.

Zinkler, M., Gaglia, A., Arokiadass, S.M.R., Farhy, E. (2007). Dialectical behaviour treatment: implementation and outcomes. *Psychiat. Bull.*, **31** 249–52.

Chapter 10

Pharmacological approaches

> **Key points**
>
> - The use of some psychotropic medications in those who are suicidal has been controversial.
> - If there is a mental disorder for which there is evidence of effective pharmacological treatment, then that treatment should be offered.
> - There are persuasive studies demonstrating the effectiveness of antidepressant, mood stabilizer and anti-psychotic medications in reducing suicidality, including suicide, in patients with mood and schizophrenic disorders.

10.1 Concerns about pharmacotherapy

At the outset it is acknowledged that at times some have expressed concern about the role of psychotropic medication in the management of those who are suicidal. Indeed, the question has even been posed as to whether such medication, apart from neuroleptics for psychotic illnesses, should be prescribed for those under the age of 40 years. Even stronger views have been expressed about the pharmacological treatment of suicidal children and adolescents.

These concerns are for several reasons. Interpersonal and family problems may appear to be medicalized; there is the risk of using medication for further suicidal behaviour; and there have been reports that antidepressants could precipitate suicidal behaviour, particularly in young persons. These concerns can be readily addressed.

Medication should only be prescribed if clinically indicated for a specific mental disorder, and suicidal behaviour per se is not an indication; it is accepted that the risk of further suicidal behaviour is ever present, and the safest medications should be prescribed in treating any underlying mental disorder which is contributing to the suicidal risk; and, with regard to the possibility of antidepressants precipitating suicidal behaviour, a number of large pharmaco-epidemiological studies have provided re-assuring results.

Put simply, if suicidal behaviour is associated with a mental disorder for which there is good evidence that a pharmacological treatment is effective, then that treatment should be offered. Naturally that is concurrent with emotional support, which may be one of the psychotherapies previously described, along with monitoring of the medication during follow-up consultations, with due regard for compliance and potential side-effects.

10.2 **Potential benefits of pharmacotherapy**

Historically it has been assumed that by treating mental disorders associated with suicide, suicidal behaviours would be reduced. In the early 1970s in the UK it was observed that as many as a fifth of suicides could have been prescribed lithium because of their recurrent affective disorders, and Swiss research two decades later reported that a significantly higher proportion of a control group, compared to 64 former psychiatric patients who had died by suicide, had been receiving psychotropic drugs, including lithium. Furthermore, a study from New York found that only 16.4% of 1,635 people who had died by suicide were on psychotropic medication, and it was observed that it was unexpected that there had not been more standard prescription psychotropic drugs used at the time of death, bearing in mind the known association between mental disorders and suicide. Similar findings were later reported from Finland, Sweden and Switzerland.

These general studies have been supplemented by more specific studies involving antidepressant, mood stabilizer, and antipsychotic medications.

10.3 **Antidepressants**

10.3.1 **Randomized Controlled Trial (RCT) evidence**
Because of the low base rate of suicide it is not feasible to mount RCTs to demonstrate a reduction in suicide per se. However, RCTs of antidepressants versus placebo have demonstrated statistically significant reductions in suicidal ideation.

Meta-analytic studies of antidepressants versus placebo have demonstrated a weak association (about one in 700) between antidepressants and nonfatal deliberate self-harm, but not suicide. This association is not specific to the newer antidepressants, with similar effects being found with tricyclic antidepressants. The jury is still out as to whether this is an idiosyncratic response, whether it is related to akathisia-like symptoms, or whether it is an artefact, as trials included in these meta-analyses were not designed to assess suicidal behaviours, and it is reasonable to consider whether suicidal behaviour with an active substance would be more likely than a placebo to be reported as an adverse event. It is also thought provoking that emerging suicidality similar to that reported in drug trials has been described in non-pharmacological psychotherapy treatment of depressed adolescents, and for almost 200 years there have been reports of unexpected suicides during the early natural history convalescence from depression.

10.3.2 Pharmaco-epidemiological studies

Probably the most persuasive data have come from large population studies. A programme to enhance the recognition and treatment of depression by general practitioners on the Swedish island of Gotland was followed by a decrease in suicide, a greater use of antidepressants, a decreased prescription of neuroleptics and hypnotics, a decrease in in-patient treatment of depression, and a reduction in sick leave due to depression. Further important work has emerged from Sweden, where a naturalistic experiment was made possible by the fact that antidepressant prescribing increased threefold, and was associated with a reduction in suicide. Similar associations were found in the other Nordic countries, and this was hailed as a 'medical break through' in suicide prevention.

Similar findings have been reported from other countries, and a comprehensive review of suicide and selective serotonin re-uptake inhibitor (SSRI) antidepressant prescribing from 27 countries reported that suicide rates fell fastest in those countries that experienced the most rapid rate of growth of SSRI scales; that a 13% increase in SSRIs was associated with a 2.5% reduction in suicide rates; and that the suicide rates in 1999 would have been 17% higher than 1990, but for the introduction of the SSRIs. However, it was also noted that the relationship was more pronounced for adults than for children.

There is less evidence for the effectiveness of antidepressants in children and adolescents than there is for adults. Nevertheless, pharmaco-epidemiological data of their suicide prevention potential has been reported from the United States, where a significant negative relationship between antidepressant treatment and suicide in different regions was found. It was calculated that a 1% increase in adolescent use of antidepressants was associated with a decrease of 0.23 suicides per 100,000 adolescents each year.

Such findings for the effectiveness of measures to treat depression having an impact on suicide are not unexpected in view of the clinical risk factors described previously, particularly those delineated by population attributable risk analyses. However, it has only been by large population studies, rather than by randomized controlled trials, that the impact on suicide has been demonstrated.

Despite the strength of these studies, they have not convinced all who have been concerned about reports of suicidal behaviour being precipitated by the newer SSRI antidepressants, particularly in the young. Notwithstanding the previously noted caveats about the data, if one accepts that there is a risk of suicidal behaviour in approximately one in 700 persons, then that needs to be balanced against the benefits of treatment. It has been estimated that between four and seven people need to be treated with the SSRI fluoxetine to give a response defined as both self and clinician report of much or very much improved, and these figures of risk and benefit can be discussed with patients in making an informed decision about treatment. Although the risk-benefit ratio is less favourable for young persons, the potential benefits of antidepressant use are not only accepted, but usually emphasized by most clinicians, rather than not using an effective treatment.

Recent research has further allayed these concerns in an emphatic manner. Five studies from the UK, Denmark, Sweden, and the United States have examined the use of SSRIs in association with suicide in young persons. In combining the data from these studies, and bearing in mind the prevalence of depression in association with suicide in the young, it was striking that only one out of 194 young suicides had evidence of SSRI use in association with their death. Such a finding is totally incongruent with the assertion that SSRI antidepressants are likely to precipitate suicide, but it is consistent with other studies that have demonstrated inadequate recognition and treatment of depression in those who die by suicide, no matter what their age.

Table 10.1 **SSRI use in young persons who died by suicide**				
Researchers	Country	Ages (yrs)	No. of suicides	SSRI anti-depressants before suicide
Jick et al (2004)	U.K.	10–19	15	0
Isacsson et al (2005)	Sweden	<15	52	0
Moskos et al (2005)	US	13–21	49	0
Sondergard et al (2006)	Denmark	10–17	42	0
Leon et al (2006)	US	<18	36	1
Total			194	1

When antidepressants are used, it is imperative that an adequate dose be prescribed. It is also essential to be aware not only of the possible risk of suicide but of the potential risk of not treating those who are depressed and suicidal.

Newer antidepressants should be prescribed because they are less toxic in overdose. It is also important that the duration of treatment is adequate. Antidepressants should be used for four to six months in patients with a first episode of major depression; for 18 to 24 months in those with a second episode; and long term on a maintenance basis in those who have had three or more episodes.

- High prevalence of mental disorders in association with suicide
- Evidence of less than expected use of medication by those who die by suicide
- RCT evidence of reduction of suicidal ideation with antidepressants
- Pharmaco-epidemiological evidence of the effectiveness of SSRI antidepressants, the mood stabilizer lithium, and the antipsychotic, clozapine in reducing suicide.

10.4 Mood stabilizers

10.4.1 Lithium

Following the previously noted UK observations in the 1970s, a number of studies have reported a reduction in suicide with consistent use of lithium in patients with affective disorders. Naturalistic observations of 1.5, 1.3 and 0.7 suicides per thousand patient years in three studies of persons on long-term lithium treatment were markedly lower than the estimated 5.1 to 11.6 suicides per thousand patient years in untreated unipolar and bipolar illnesses. More recent reviews have added weight to these reports. A meta-analysis of 31 studies with patients having 85,229 person years of risk exposure concluded that the overall risk of suicide and attempted suicide was five times less among lithium treated patients than those not treated with lithium. It has also been reported that although lithium probably prevents about 250 suicides per year in Germany, only 0.06% of the German population were prescribed lithium, and that even if one assumed both a conservative estimate of the prevalence of bipolar disorders and that only half would be prescribed lithium, then rational treatment would dictate that prescription rates of lithium should be approximately ten times higher.

10.4.2 Anticonvulsants

The question of whether or not anticonvulsant mood stabilizers have suicide protective qualities similar to those of lithium has been addressed in a retrospective cohort study of 20,638 health plan members with bipolar disorder. Suicide and suicide attempts were 2.7 and 1.7 times respectively higher with sodium valproate compared to lithium treatment, a statistically significant finding. Another study examining lithium, carbamazepine and amitriptyline in mood disorders in 378 subjects over a 2.5 year period reported that of the five suicide attempts and nine suicides, none had occurred during lithium treatment, and a further study reported that lamotrigine also had no effect on suicidality.

None of these studies involved randomized controlled trials, but the results are compelling, with the best available evidence at present being that the mood stabilizer of choice for bipolar disorders with suicidality is lithium. Naturally this choice needs to be weighed up with regard to tolerability of side effects, compliance issues in regard to monitoring, and patient acceptance.

10.5 Antipsychotic (neuroleptic) medication

There had been a sense of pessimism about schizophrenia and suicide until observations in the mid 90s in the United States that neuroleptic resistant patients treated with clozapine for between six months and seven years (mean 3.5 years) had 'markedly less suicidality' than non-clozapine treated patients. Attempted suicide decreased from 25% to 3.5%; the lethality of suicide attempts which did occur was reduced; suicidal intent was reduced; and there was a significant decrease in hopelessness. Subsequently it was reported that of 102,000 patients treated for schizophrenia with clozapine there were 39 suicides, with a rate adjusted for duration of treatment of 0.1% to 0.2% per year, which is about one quarter of the rate one would anticipate on the basis of previous follow-up studies of those with schizophrenia. There were similar findings from another American study of 30,000 patients with schizophrenia and schizoaffective disorder, with clozapine treated patients having a suicide rate of 12.7 per 100,000 per year compared to the 63.1 per 100,000 per year for all patients with those disorders in the United States.

These findings led to the establishment of an ambitious multi-centre trial in 67 centres in 11 countries comparing clozapine with the atypical antipsychotic olanzapine. A total of 980 patients with schizophrenia or schizo-affective disorder were randomized to the treatments and non-pharmacological input was identical. Clozapine was significantly more effective in reducing suicide attempts, hospitalisation and the need for emergency intervention, but the suicides were too few for statistical analysis. It was evident that clozapine was more effective than olanzapine, regardless of any individual risk factor such as substance abuse or number of previous suicide attempts.

As clozapine is usually reserved for those with resistance to conventional antipsychotic medication, these results are particularly persuasive. Although olanzapine was not as effective in terms of reduction of suicidality as clozapine in those severely ill patients, it has been reported to reduce suicide attempts when compared to haloperidol treated patients. Post-marketing surveillance reports suggest that the atypical antipsychotics quetiapine and risperidone have reduced suicidality compared to the typical antipsychotic haloperidol. However, it can not be assumed that the newer atypical antipsychotics as a whole (except clozapine) are more effective in reducing suicidality than the older medications, as in the large Clinical Antipsychotic Trials of Intervention Effectiveness (CATIE) study there were no differences in suicide attempts or suicidal ideation reported as adverse events between the atypical antipsychotics olanzapine, quetiapine, risperidone and ziprasidone compared to the typical antipsychotic perphenazine. Nevertheless, there is now more reason to believe that vigorous treatment of schizophrenia, particularly with clozapine, has the potential to reduce the likelihood of suicidal behaviours.

10.6 **Compliance**

If compliance with medication is an issue, consideration should be given to using treatment or Guardianship Board orders appropriate to the local community. By the time such approaches are necessary, community mental health workers are likely to be involved. However, it is still important for each patient to have a family practitioner who co-ordinates overall management, particularly in this era of deinstitutionalization. The family practitioner is in a good position to provide continuity of care, which is at a premium in some public health systems.

10.7 **Rationale for pharmacological treatment**

It should be re-iterated that medications are prescribed not specifically to prevent suicide, but to treat the mental disorders associated with suicidal behaviour. They are simply one component of the standard care which should be provided by a modern health service.

References

Angst, F., Stassen, H.H., Clayton, P.J., Angst, J. (2002). Mortality of patients with mood disorders: Follow-up over 34–38 years. *J. Aff. Dis.*, **68**, 167–81.

Baldessarini, R.J., Tondo, L., Davis, P. *et al.* (2006). Dereased risk of suicides and attempts during long-term lithium treatment: a meta-analytic review. *Bipolar Disord.*, **8**, 625–39.

Barraclough, B. (1972). Suicide prevention, recurrent affective disorder and lithium. *Br. J. Psychiat.*, **121**, 391–2.

Bridge, J.A., Barbe, R.P., Birmaher, B. *et al.* (2005). Emergent suicidality in a clinical psychotherapy trial for adolescent depression. *Am. J. Psychiat.*, **162**, 2173–5.

Goldney, R.D. (2007). Antidepressants and suicide in young people. *Med. J. Aust.*, **187**, 586–7.

Goodwin, F.K., Fireman, B., Simon, G.E. *et al.* (2003). Suicide risk in bipolar disorders during treatment with lithium and divalproex. *J.A.M.A.*, **290**, 1467–73.

Gunnell, D, Saperia, J., Ashby, D. (2007). Selective serotonin reuptake inhibitors (SSRIs) and suicide in adults: meta-analysis of drug company data from placebo controlled, randomised controlled trials submitted to the MHRA's safety review. *B.M.J.*, **330**, 385–9.

Isacsson, G. (2002). Suicide prevention—a medical break-through? *Acta Psychiat. Scand.*, **102**, 113–17.

Isacsson, G., Holmgren, P., Ahlner, J. (2005). Selective serotonin reuptake inhibitor antidepressants and the risk of suicide: a controlled forensic database study of 14857 suicides. *Acta Psychiat. Scand.*, **111**, 286–90.

Jick, H., Kaye, J.A., Jick, S.S. (2004). Antidepressants and the risk of suicidal behaviours. *J.A.M.A.*, **292**, 338–43.

Leon, A.C., Marzuk, P.M., Tardiff, K. *et al.* (2006). Antidepressants and Youth Suicide in New York City. *J. Am. Acad. Child Adolesc. Psychiat.*, **45**, 1054–8.

Letizia, C., Kapik, B., Flanders, W.D. (1996). Suicidal risk during controlled clinical investigations of Fluvoxamine. *J. Clin. Psychiat.*, **57**, 415–21.

Ludwig, J., Marcotte, D.E. (2005). Anti-depressants, suicide, and drug regulation. *J. Policy Anal. Manage.*, **24**, 249–72.

Marzuk, P.M., Tardiff, K., Leon, A.C., *et al.* (1995). Use of prescription psychotropic drugs among suicide victims in New York City. *Am. J. Psychiat.* **152**, 1520–22.

Meltzer, H.Y., Okayli, G. (1995). Reduction of suicidality during clozapine treatment of neuroleptic-resistant schizophrenia: Impact on risk benefit assessment. *Am. J. Psychiat.*, **152**, 183–90.

Meltzer, H.Y., Alphs, L., Green, A.I., *et al.* (2003). Clozapine treatment for suicidality in schizophrenia. International Suicide Prevention Trial (InterSePT). *Arch. Gen. Psychiat.*, **60**, 82–91.

Moskos, M., Olson, L., Halbern, S. *et al.* (2005). Utah youth suicide study: psychological autopsy. *Suicide Life threat. Behav.*, **35**, 536–46.

Muller-Oerlinghausen, B., Felber, W., Berghofer, A. (2005). The impact of lithium long-term medication on suicidal behaviour and mortality of bipolar patients. *Arch. Sui. Res.*, **9**, 307–19.

Olfson, M., Shaffer, D., Marcus, S.C., Greenberg, T. (2003). Relationship between antidepressant medication treatment and suicide in adolescents. *Arch. Gen. Psychiat.*, **60**, 978–82.

Oquendo, M., Chaudhury, S.R., Mann, J.J. (2005). Pharmacotherapy of suicidal behavior in bipolar disorder. *Arch. Sui. Res.*, **9**, 237–50.

Reid, W.H., Mason, M., Hogan, T. (1998). Suicide prevention effects associated with clozapine therapy in schizophrenia and schizoaffective disorder. *Psychiat. Serv.*, **49**, 1029–33.

Rutz, W., von Knorring, L., Walinder, J. (1992). Long-term effects of an educational program for general practitioners given by the Swedish Committee for the prevention and treatment of depression. *Acta Psychiat. Scand.*, **85**, 83–8.

Sondergard, L., Kvist, K., Andersen, P.K. *et al.* (2006). Do antidepressants precipitate youth suicide? A nationwide pharmacoepidemiological study. *Europ. Child Adolesc. Psychiat.*, **15**, 232–40.

Szanto, K., Mulsant, B.H., Houck, P., Dew, M.A., Reynolds, C.F. (2003). Occurrence and course of suicidality during short-term treatment of late-life depression. *Archs. Gen. Psychiat.*, **60**, 610–17.

Chapter 11

Broad suicide prevention initiatives

> **Key points**
> - Many of the longitudinal antecedents of suicide are important social issues in their own right
> - Restriction of access to means of suicide is effective and usually requires political will and legislation to introduce
> - Responsible media reporting favourably influences suicide rates
> - National programmes of suicide prevention are associated with a reduction in suicide
> - More focussed community initiatives have also been effective.

11.1 Limitations of the individual approach

It will be evident from a consideration of the diverse contributing factors to suicide that the individual clinician has only limited options at his or her disposal in managing suicidal behaviour. These options necessarily include the comprehensive clinical evaluation of those who may be suicidal, and the implementation of standard management practices, as described.

11.2 Lobbying for action

While other options may appear to be limited, it is important to lobby for change in regard to the broader and at times more distal contributing factors. These include child abuse, particularly sexual abuse; other family violence; community safety nets such as adequate pensions and general health care; safety in custody and in prisons; indigenous rights; homophobia; bullying in schools and the work place; and general stigma about mental disorders and equity of access for their management. However, each of these issues is important in its own right, and the remote possibility of suicide is hardly a compelling reason to urge legislators to act, even though it is often used emotionally as a device to seek publicity and demand action. Nevertheless, by addressing such factors governments are seen to be caring, and long term benefits should ensue, even though it may not be possible to devise research methodologies to clinch what may have been the precise effective component.

Broad approaches with the potential for more immediate results include the restriction of access to means of suicide and modification of the reporting of suicide by the media.

11.3 **Restriction of access to means of suicide**

This public health approach provides persuasive data illustrating that legislative measures to restrict access to the means of suicide are effective. The reduction in suicide due to barbiturate poisoning in Australia following the blister packaging of medication and restriction on the number of tablets/capsules prescribed was probably the first convincing example. This was followed by what has come to be known as 'The coal gas story' in the UK, where the introduction of non-toxic North Sea gas resulted in a sustained reduction in suicide of about 30%. This was associated with a modest increase in suicide by other means, particularly in the younger age groups, but that increase was relatively small, and it was masked by the overall reduction, particularly as suicide by coal gas had been a preferred method of suicide in the UK.

Since then there have been reports of the effectiveness of barriers on jumping sites, such as bridges and car parks. Furthermore, there was a 22% reduction in suicide deaths due to paracetamol in the year following legislation to restrict the availability of analgesics in England and Wales. That reduction was sustained in the subsequent two years, and there was also a 30% reduction in the need for liver transplants due to paracetamol induced hepatotoxicity.

In developing countries the ready availability of highly lethal pesticides is being addressed, and in Sri Lanka the suicide rate has almost halved from 47 per 100,000 in 1995 to 24 per 100,000 in 2005, following legislation in 1995 and 1998 to restrict the import and sale of toxic pesticides. There was a reduction in suicide in all ages, in both men and women, and there were 19,769 fewer suicides in the period 1996–2005 compared with 1986–1995. Naturally it is too simplistic to state that the restrictive legislation was the only factor in reducing suicide, as other measures such as enhancing clinical services and the impact of volunteer organizations would have played a role as well. Nevertheless, it is probable that this dramatic reduction has been related predominantly to the restriction of access to a very lethal means of suicide.

Firearms are the most common cause of suicide in the United States, and although there is unequivocal case-control evidence of an association between the possession of firearms in a household and an increased risk of suicide, the American belief in the right to bear arms is a stumbling block to legislative change. However, in those regions where there has been restrictive legislation, there has been an associated reduction in suicide, and that has also been demonstrated in a number of other countries including Canada, Australia, New Zealand and Austria. Furthermore, a case-control study has demonstrated that storing a firearm in a locked location; storing it unloaded; ensuring the ammunition is locked; and storing the ammunition separately, are each associated with a protective effect.

> **Box 11.1 Effective restriction of access to means of suicide**
>
> - Barbiturate prescribing legislation
> - 'The coal gas story'
> - Barriers to jumping – bridges, car parks
> - Restriction of availability of pesticides
> - Paracetamol prescribing legislation
> - Firearms restriction legislation.

Carbon monoxide poisoning by motor vehicle is a major method of suicide in some countries and potentially preventable. Catalytic converters have minimized the risk, but baffles could be manufactured into exhaust systems, and a sensor could be placed inside the cabin to immobilize the engine when carbon monoxide was detected. While such measures are hardly likely to be part of a motor vehicle manufacturer's advertising spiel, they could be legislated for if there was sufficient community pressure.

Hanging is the most common form of suicide in some countries and the means are widely available and not subject to potential legislation. Only about 20% occur in controlled environments such as prisons or hospitals, thereby limiting the opportunity for intervention. Nevertheless, potential hanging sites should be eliminated in custodial and treatment settings.

The restriction of access to means is probably effective not only because of the preclusion of a lethal method of suicide per se, but also because it buys time, as the final suicidal impulse nearly always dissipates with time. It is also important to emphasize that most of these public health initiatives to reduce access to means of suicide require legislation and the political will to introduce them.

11.4 Modification of media reporting

There is unequivocal evidence that indiscriminate reporting of suicidal behaviour is associated with increases in suicide, and yet the media are courted to promulgate suicide prevention initiatives. This presents a dilemma: how does one balance the freedom of the press with social responsibility? This question has led to co-operation with media representatives, and guidelines for responsible reporting about suicide have been developed. These are along the lines of not sensationalizing reporting by providing lurid details; not having suicide as front page news; not idealizing those who die by suicide; reporting that suicide is usually associated with a remediable mental health problem; and emphasizing that there are more appropriate alternatives.

That co-operation with the media does have an effect on reporting was demonstrated by an analysis of newspapers in Switzerland after the provision of guidelines, where the percentage of suicides being front page news reduced from 20% to 4%, and sensational headlines reduced from 62% to 25%.

One of the first examples of effective suicide prevention by such an approach was in Vienna, where responsible reporting of subway suicides resulted in the number of suicides reducing by 70%. Other studies from Austria have also reported a favourable impact of media guidelines, with there being a significant reduction in suicide in regions with the highest coverage rate of collaborating newspapers. Indeed, for one specific celebrity suicide the dose-response effect of regional differences in reporting explained 40% of the variance of change in the numbers of those dying by suicide.

While it is evident that responsible reporting can minimize the adverse effect of media publicity, the question should be asked as to whether the media may have a positive impact on general suicide rates. Volunteer organizations such as the Samaritans and other Crisis centres rely on media publicity, as do some mental health education programmes, but reductions in suicidal behaviour as a result of specifically designed media/publicity campaigns have yet to be demonstrated.

11.5 National programmes

Governments were slow to appreciate the enormous impact of suicidal behaviour, not only at the individual human level, but also on the broader economic cost at the population level. The first National approach was in 1985, when Finnish health authorities inaugurated a programme to lower the suicide rate by 20% over the next ten years. In fact, suicide increased initially, but then reduced to a figure about 9% below the initial level. The programme was research based and involved community education about risk factors, with guidebooks for health promotion provided for schools, the armed services, and clergy, as well as the Social Services sector. In an evaluation it was acknowledged that there had been gaps between the medical model and socio-cultural paradigms in understanding and preventing suicidal behaviour, and it was thought that more attention could have been paid to reducing access to means of suicide and to suicide prevention in the elderly. Nevertheless, it was considered that the project did contribute to the reduction in suicide rate.

A number of other countries have since introduced national programmes, all of which have certain similarities. An example is the United States strategy, which was launched in 2001. Its 'Goals and Objectives for Action' were:

1. Promote awareness that suicide is a public health problem that is preventable
2. Develop broad-based support for suicide prevention
3. Develop and implement strategies to reduce the stigma associated with being a consumer of mental health, substance abuse and suicide prevention services
4. Develop and implement community-based suicide prevention programs
5. Promote efforts to reduce access to lethal means and methods of self-harm
6. Implement training for recognition of at-risk behavior and delivery of effective treatment
7. Develop and promote effective clinical and professional practices
8. Increase access to and community linkages with mental health and substance abuse services
9. Improve reporting and portrayals of suicidal behavior, mental illness and substance abuse in the entertainment and news media
10. Promote and support research on suicide and suicide prevention
11. Improve and expand surveillance systems.

It is apparent that these goals and objectives include most aspects of suicide prevention and research, and it is reassuring that there have been reductions in suicide not only in the United States, but also in those other countries which have embraced such wide reaching programmes. For example, the suicide rate in Australia reduced by almost 30% from its peak in 1997 to 2004, and there was a reduction of about 50% in young males aged 15 to 24 years. Debate has arisen about what may have been the specific effective component of the change, and one study concluded that improved detection and management of depression may have played a role. However, the complexity of determining the exact reason for that reduction in suicide is demonstrated well by the sobering observation that the change in young males was confined to the middle and higher socio-economic groups, and the historical predominance of rural suicides actually increased. Clearly the broad programme in Australia did not reach certain groups in the community, even though the overall impact was positive.

National interventions can be criticized for their general nature and the lack of specific theoretical framework. However, there have been two recent reports of large scale community interventions which have been more focussed and rigorous in their research design, and which have produced encouraging results.

11.6 **More focussed community interventions**

Following the introduction of a community based programme to a cohort of over five million United States Air Force personnel, there was a reduction of 33% in suicide between 1990–1996 and 1997–2002. The programme focussed on the removal of stigma from seeking help for psychosocial problems, enhancing mental health literacy, and changing administrative policies to facilitate access to intervention services. It is also important that there were reductions in accidental death, homicide, and family violence, which is not unexpected as they share many of the antecedents of suicidal behaviours.

Positive results have also been reported from Germany in the Nuremberg Alliance against Depression study, where a two year campaign to inform people about depression, train family doctors, encourage co-operation with community facilitators such as teachers, priests and the media, and also support self-help groups, resulted in a statistically significant reduction in suicidal acts in Nuremberg compared to Wuerzburg, which did not participate in the programme and was used as a control region.

11.7 **Conclusion**

Broad community interventions are challenging to evaluate, and those who demand RCT evidence are unlikely to be satisfied by their results, no matter how much face validity they may possess. Potentially effective individual components are difficult to tease out, but this is being addressed by increasingly sophisticated non-RCT research methodologies. These have given confidence that the broad approaches described are effective. However, it is important that clinicians do not pursue lobbying for such programmes at the expense of careful assessment and management of the individual suicidal person.

References

Etzersdorfer, E., Voracek, M., Sonneck, G. (2004). A dose-response relationship between imitational suicides and newspaper distribution. *Arch. Suicide Res.*, **8**, 137–45.

Goldney, R.D. (2006). Suicide in Australia: Some good news. *Med. J. Aust.*, **185**, 304.

Gunnell, D., Bennewith, O., Hawton, K. *et al.* (2005). The epidemiology and prevention of suicide by hanging: a systematic review. *Int. J. Epidemiol.*, **34**. 433–42.

Hegerl, U., Althaus, D., Schmidtke, A., Niklewski, G. (2006). The alliance against depression: 2-year evaluation of a community-based intervention to reduce suicidality. *Psychol. Med.*, **36**, 1225–33.

Knox, K.L., Litts, D.A., Talcott, G.W. *et al.* (2003). Risk of suicide and related adverse outcomes after exposure to a suicide prevention programme in the US Air Force: Cohort study. *B. Med. J.*, **327**, 1376–80.

Kreitman, N. (1976). The coal gas story. *Br. J. Prev. Soc. Med.*, **30**, 86–93.

Michel, K., Frey, C., Wyss, K., Valach, L. (2000). An exercise in improving suicide reporting in print media. *Crisis*, **21**, 71–9.

Niederkrotenthaler, T., Sonneck, G. (2007). Assessing the impact of media guidelines for reporting on suicides in Austria: interrupted time series analysis. *Aust. N.Z. J. Psychiat.*, **41**, 419–28.

U.S. Department of Health and Human Services. (2001). National Strategy for Suicide Prevention: Goals and Objectives for Action. Public Health Service, Rockville, MD.

Chapter 12

Bereavement after suicide

> ## Key points
>
> - There are qualitative differences in grief themes in those bereaved through suicide
> - Themes include shock; disbelief; horror; how?; why?; guilt and blame; relief vs. family disaster; rejection; stigma, shame and social isolation; a wasted life; suicidal thoughts and fear of another suicide; and anger
> - Practical issues include viewing the body and having sensitive funeral arrangements
> - Therapists are vulnerable to similar feelings in addition to concerns about their professional competence.

For every death by suicide approximately six people suffer intense grief, leading to there being as many as six million people worldwide each year who are bereaved through suicide. Traditionally, suicide has been regarded as being associated with complicated grief, and early case studies described major pathology among relatives and friends. However, the use of more rigorous methodologies, with comparison groups such as those bereaved through accidental death, with more sophisticated data analysis, including control for sociodemographic variables, has modified this opinion. Indeed, recent reviewers have concluded that the previously held belief that suicide bereavement was more severe cannot be supported.

12.1 Qualitative differences from other bereavement

The present consensus is that there are more similarities than differences in morbidity between those bereaved through suicide and through other causes, and the specific mode of death itself creates few if any quantitative differences in bereavement outcome, although recovery may be slower in the first two years after a suicide. However, there are differences in the themes of grief. It is also possible that the 'crisis atmosphere' which often surrounds suicide may lead to stigmatizing views about suicide bereavement.

Recent studies have found that better predictors of bereavement outcome than the mode of death include: the age of the deceased; the kinship lost; the age, gender and culture of the bereaved; their attitude to the loss; and the quality of their relationship with the deceased. Thus parents of young adults with whom they have had a difficult relationship, and who perceive there to be inadequate support in their grief, are most at risk.

Suicide often occurs in an already psychosocially burdened family, with a higher prevalence of psychiatric illness and there may be inter-generational effects. Indeed, contrary to some earlier views, suicidal behaviour does run in some families, and therefore those bereaved by suicide are an 'at-risk' group, not so much because of the mode of death itself, but because suicide identifies the vulnerable.

12.2 Grief themes

There are certain commonalities to emotional experiences following suicide. An understanding of these themes has come from qualitative studies, and in clinical practice it is useful to address them albeit with an appreciation that they are not discrete but overlapping in nature, and that there is no set time-table for their emergence. These include:

Table 12.1 Grief themes in bereavement through suicide	
• Shock	• Relief vs family disaster
• Disbelief	• Rejection
• Horror	• Stigma, shame and isolation
• How?	• A wasted life
• Why?	• Suicidal thoughts and fear of another suicide
• Guilt and blame	• Anger

12.2.1 Shock
The shock of discovering the deceased may be recurring and long-lasting, with flash backs of discovering the body, or experiences of feelings and smells associated with cleaning up residue of the deceased.

12.2.2 Disbelief
Disbelief may be overwhelming and the bereaved may cling to other explanations for the death. Such convictions may be reinforced by feelings of shame, so that false information about the cause of death may be given.

12.2.3 Horror
The feeling of horror may include the realization of the extreme depth of distress the deceased must have been in. The bereaved may fantasize about the suffering of the dying process and, if it was slow, whether the deceased had changed his/her mind, but was too late to act.

12.2.4 **How?**

The family may wish to know precisely how the person died, whether drugs or medications were ingested, and the physical and mental effects of those substances. A sensitive interpretation of the post mortem report or coronial enquiry may assist.

12.2.5 **Why?**

This is probably the most common theme in bereavement after suicide, and ultimately there is no satisfactory answer. Questions arise about what external pressures were acting on the deceased, and why there was a breakdown in communication in regard to seeking help. A suicide note may influence the bereaved into assuming responsibility and guilt. Blame from others may be experienced.

12.2.6 **Guilt and blame**

Guilt and blame commonly arise from the quest for 'why?'. The bereaved may feel they contributed to the suicide and blame themselves for not having prevented it. Parents may feel there was something suspect in their parenting. They may feel that as the closest in kinship to their child, they should have been the ones to see the signs of hopelessness and to have acted as their child's confidante. 'If only …' is a common phrase used to describe acts which might have prevented the suicide. Some families feel they did all they could, whereas others, even if they had participated in the deceased's care, may have unrealistic feelings of remorse. Guilt may also be felt at the sense of relief created by the death.

12.2.7 **Relief vs. family disaster**

For some families the suicide becomes a means of resolving existing problems and threats, whereas for others it is clearly a disaster. Families who struggle for years with a depressed individual and suicidal threats may experience relief, as their family life has an opportunity to return to normal. Indeed, suicide may have been regarded as inevitable, following the deterioration in mental state of the distressed person. By the time suicide occurs, the family may have accepted mental illness as the cause of death, and by so doing, feelings of guilt, shame, and rejection may be reduced. They may also be comforted that the deceased is out of distress, even though they regret the means.

On the other hand, for some families the suicide creates disaster. This includes families who had previously regarded themselves as functioning normally, and the suicide has been quite unexpected. For already disadvantaged families, with limited problem solving ability, the suicide adds to their problems and increases dysfunction.

12.2.8 **Rejection**

Suicide is sometimes felt as a conscious rejection of the family, and following difficult relationships they may interpret the death as a malicious act with no opportunity for redress. The bereaved are in essence the victims of the omnipotent mastery of the deceased.

12.2.9 **Stigma, shame, and social isolation**

Feelings of stigma vary between studies and appear to be culturally-based. Even where stigma is absent, feelings of shame may arise due to guilt, blame, rejection, being the subject of gossip, and the association of suicide with mental disorders. Some families feel there is a tainting of the family tree, or come to hold superstitious beliefs that the suicide was caused by evil in the family.

Shame plays an important role in constraining interpersonal relationships and the bereaved may create their own social isolation. There may also be a lack of emotional support for those bereaved through suicide, and community studies indicate a mismatch in knowledge and attitudes between the bereaved and professional or community groups. After suicide the bereaved may have the additional burden of educating their friends about the causes and nature of suicide and about how to behave toward them.

12.2.10 **A wasted life**

Remorse at the waste of a life and at the unfulfillable opportunities for the deceased person and for members of the bereaved family are common themes.

12.2.11 **Suicidal thoughts and fear of another suicide**

Suicidal thoughts are common and may be in part a longing to rejoin the deceased and to complete unfinished business, or it can be associated with depression. Added fears about a repeat family suicide may result in families becoming over-protective; in particular, parents may worry about the risk to younger siblings when they reach the age at which the older child took his/her life. Adolescents may have difficulty dealing with the boundaries between themselves and a role model who took his/her life, or even feel fated to die. Acquaintances may worry about contagion, which may cause them to withdraw support.

12.2.12 **Anger**

Anger at the deceased may result from the emotional pain experienced, particularly if the bereaved person was blamed in a suicide note, or offered help and had been rejected. When a partner suicides there may be anger at being cheated out of the relationship or at being left to carry the full burden of the family's responsibilities. Anger may also be expressed towards the health care team, God or the therapist, or towards the press for inaccurate, exaggerated or sensational reports, and for the loss of privacy at the time of family tragedy.

12.3 Practical issues and bereavement care

A physician certifying death at the site of a suicide can allay initial confusion and provide explanation about such matters as why resuscitation was stopped, or not begun, and the need for official investigation at a time of personal tragedy. It is important to be honest about the cause of death, as that will prevent difficulties in trying to maintain future deceptions.

Opportunity should be offered to view the body, but if it is mutilated the alternative of maintaining vigil over the covered body may be preferred. Families may be angry if this opportunity is denied. If a decision is taken not to view the body, negotiations should be made with a family member or the funeral director to take photographs of the body in case of future need. These may be useful later to alleviate fantasies of misidentification or trauma in the dying process.

If a public funeral is not held, regrets about not giving adequate tribute to the deceased may arise. In addition, the opportunity is denied for other significant mourners, such as school friends or work colleagues, to grieve. If the funeral is private or if there is no funeral at all, the bereaved may also deprive themselves of the usual demonstrations of support.

An explanation of various models of suicide, particularly the biological model, may be helpful in understanding why the deceased took his/her life, and such a no-blame model may alleviate feelings of guilt, rejection, and shame. Any apparent social stress or other environmental causes of the suicide must, of course, be acknowledged. Explanation of the impossibility of prediction of suicide in any individual, even by professionals, may assist in allaying concerns that the bereaved should have prevented the suicide.

Counselling may be helpful to assist a bereaved person to rationalize unrealistic feelings, particularly guilt, rejection, and those arising from the suicide note. A gentle exploration of feelings, on the basis that the introjection of such feelings contributes to emotional distress, is usually therapeutic, although the timing of such intervention needs judgement. Antidepressant or other psychotropic medications may be utilized if indicated as an adjunct to the psychological grief work, rather than as a replacement for it. The quest for why the suicide occurred may become all-consuming, and directing the bereaved to turn their attention to other grief themes and here and now issues will be more productive.

In some communities support groups have developed for those bereaved by suicide. They are valuable for some in assisting bereaved persons to recognize that their feelings of intense emotional pain are normal, and to provide experiential expertise and role models of survival. Other important functions are those of advocacy within the community and destigmatization.

12.4 The therapist's reaction

The therapist's own response to suicide has recently received attention, and sequelae have been described in a wide range of professionals and volunteers. There are feelings of personal loss, shock, sadness, and also relief that intolerable suffering is over, and that the stress of professional vigilance has ended. There may also be feelings of professional failure, fear for one's reputation, and anger at the deceased for the disruption he/she caused. Lasting personal sequelae, such as physical sickness, depression, irrational fears, and deterioration in interpersonal and professional relationships, may also occur.

Other sequelae include depersonalization and distancing from patients and colleagues, or the opposite of over-involvement in the professional role, absenteeism, fear of anger from the family and of malpractice suits, and even change of career. Female therapists have a greater tendency to feel more shame and guilt, to doubt their professional expertise, and to seek consolation. No differences have been found according to years of experience or profession. Therapists may find themselves in the dilemma of dealing with their own emotions at the same time as being required to provide objective support to the bereaved family, fellow-patients of the suicide victim, and team members.

There exist few accounts of preparation for therapists or institutions for a suicide. Recommendations include training to deal with the personal and professional issues of the aftermath, a contingency plan and review protocol for the institution, and the availability of professional support for the individual therapist.

12.5 Conclusion

Findings from rigorous comparative studies show that bereavement through suicide is no more difficult than bereavement following other modes of death, although there are different grief themes. However, it is more likely that families bereaved through suicide are also struggling with pre-existing problems, which may complicate the grieving process. The bereaved are left with difficult emotional themes and questions which are different in many respect from those resulting from other modes of death, and which are important for professionals and carers to understand so that appropriate bereavement care can be provided.

References

Clark, S.E., Goldney, R.D. (1995). Grief reactions and recovery in a support group for people bereaved by suicide. *Crisis*, **16**, 27–33.

Cleiren, M.P.H.D., Grad, O., Zavasnik, A., Diekstra, R.F.W. (1996). Psycho-social impact of bereavement after suicide and fatal traffic accident: a comparative two-country study. *Acta Psychiat. Scan.*, **94**, 37–44.

de Groot, M., de Keijser, J., Neeleman, J., Kerkhof, et. al. (2007). Cognitive behaviour therapy to prevent complicated grief among relatives and spouses bereaved by suicide: cluster randomised controlled trial. *Br. Med. J.*, **334**, 994–6.

Farberow, N., Gallagher-Thompson, D.E., Gilewski, M., Thompson, L. (1992). The role of social supports in the bereavement process of surviving spouses of suicide and natural death. *Suicide Life-Threat. Behav.*, **22**, 107–24.

Grad, O.T., Zavasnik, A. (1996). Similarities and differences in the process of bereavement after suicide and after traffic fatalities in Slovenia. *Omega*, **33**, 245–51.

Hendin, H., Lipschitz, A., Maltsberger, J.T., et al. (2000). Therapists' reactions to patients' suicides. *Am. J. Psychiat.*, **157**, 2022–7.

Séguin, M., Lesage, A., Kiely, M.C. (1995). Parental bereavement after suicide and accident: a comparative study. *Suicide Life-Threat. Behav.* **25**, 489–98.

Chapter 13

Frequently asked questions

> **Key points**
> - Asking about suicide does not increase the risk
> - The management of younger and older persons, and also those with self-harm requires modification of the overall management approach
> - Suicide bombers should be more accurately described as homicide bombers
> - There is no evidence that no-harm contracts are effective
> - De-institutionalization may be associated with increased suicide
> - The Internet has both potential negative and positive effects on suicidal behaviour
> - Enquiries about the causes of suicide should be conducted with full awareness of the limitation of our capacity to predict suicide.

13.1 Does asking about suicidal behaviour lead to an increase in such behaviour?

This question has troubled professionals and lay persons alike, and at times it has led to the curtailing of research involving specific questions about suicidal behaviour, particularly when younger populations have been examined. Clinical experience indicates that the vast majority of those who acknowledge such behaviour feel relieved about its disclosure, but there has remained doubt as to whether those who had not been suicidal could be influenced adversely.

A recent comprehensive analysis of possible risk associated with such enquiry involved 2,342 students in six high schools in New York State. All participated in a survey, but only half received questions about suicidal behaviour and the other half did not. A measure of distress was given to all students at the beginning and end of an initial survey, and at the beginning of a second assessment two days later. The experimental and control groups did not differ on distress levels after the first survey or two days later on scores of a mood instrument.

Students who had been asked questions about suicide were no more likely to report suicidal ideation compared to the control students, and students who were considered to be at high risk with symptoms of depression, substance use problems or a past suicide attempt, were neither more suicidal nor more distressed than similar high risk youth in the control group. Indeed, it was found that those who were depressed and had had a previous suicide attempt were significantly less distressed two days after the initial assessment than high risk students in the control group, an indication that the enquiry had been of benefit.

The results of this research were consistent with the previously noted clinical observation, and they not only lend confidence to attempts to identify suicidal persons in the community by direct enquiry, but they also lay to rest the suggestion that asking about suicidal behaviour leads to an iatrogenic increased risk of suicidal behaviours.

13.2 Is management of suicidal children and adolescents different?

The role of mental disorders in the suicidal behaviour of children and adolescents is less definite than in adults and more focus needs to be placed on family and interpersonal issues. Furthermore, young children and adolescents are not the same, and there is an increasing emphasis on the delineation of substantive mental disorders throughout adolescence, beginning from puberty. Nevertheless, the general principles of management remain. Suicidal behaviour needs to be taken seriously; full assessment should be undertaken and management appropriate to the presence or absence of specific disorders needs to be instituted. For young people family involvement should occur, and cooperation with school and social service personnel may also be required.

Antidepressants are less effective for younger persons, and only fluoxetine has been approved for use in major depression in children and adolescents by regulatory authorities in the U.K. and the United States. The risk benefit ratio for the use of antidepressants for major depression in those under the age of 19 was reviewed in a meta analysis of 13 studies, and the number needed to treat for benefit was 10 whereas the number needed to treat for combined suicidal ideation/suicide attempt was 143.

Antidepressants are not the first line of treatment, as CBT involving the family should be utilized and then, if there has been no response, fluoxetine should be implemented. There is no evidence that CBT adds to the treatment effectiveness of fluoxetine and routine care of adolescents with major depression who have not responded to initial non-pharmacological interventions.

If that is not effective, then psychosocial factors need to be reviewed and, ideally, a second opinion should be sought prior to using an alternative SSRI. It is appreciated that a second opinion may not always be feasible, and it is not mandatory, particularly in view of the reassuring data in regard to the previous concern about the possibility of antidepressants precipitating suicidal behaviour in the young, as noted in Chapter 10.

13.3 Is management of self-harm different?

Self-harm arises predominantly in adolescence and the principles noted about the treatment of children and adolescents apply for those with self-harm. Thus clearly defined mental disorders are less likely to be diagnosed and therefore non-pharmacological treatments along the lines described previously will be the initial management of choice. Self-harm is often a feature of borderline personality disorder and therefore the principals of dialectical behaviour therapy are of most use in ongoing treatment.

The most persuasive data indicating that those with self-harm should be managed in a manner similar to those with what is generally regarded as a greater degree of suicidality, such as those who actually have suicidal ideation or who have attempted suicide, has been pro-vided by a follow-up study of 218,304 emergency department patients over an average period of six years, where those persons who had had a single emergency department visit for self-harm, an overdose, or suicidal ideation, had similar relative rates of subsequent suicide of 5.8, 5.7, and 6.7 times that of other emergency room attenders. Any mental disorders should be treated appropriately, and the broad principles of management are the same no matter what the age of the person who may be presenting with self-harm.

13.4 Is management of the older suicidal person different?

In contrast to young persons, suicidal behaviour in those over the age of 55 is more likely to be associated with definitely diagnosable mental disorders, almost invariably major depression, often with associated melancholia. Suicide attempts are usually of higher suicidal intent and physical lethality, and the ratio of suicide attempts to completed suicide is less. Physical treatments are more likely to be utilized, and they include not only psychotropic medication, but also electro-convulsive therapy. Newly diagnosed major depression in older persons is sometimes associated with early cerebro-vascular changes and treatments may be less effective.

Approval by family members for treatment may be required if a person's mental state is severely impaired, and in the absence of family, authorized Guardianship Boards may need to intervene to ensure that adequate treatment is provided. It is emphasized that suicidal ideation in the elderly is not an inevitable feature of old age, but an indicator of a potentially treatable depressive condition.

13.5 **Are suicide bombers suicidal?**

The term 'suicide bomber' has entered our lexicon on the obvious basis that the individual perpetrator dies. However, recent reviews have demonstrated that there is little else in common with suicidal behaviour.

From the individual psychological perspective, the usual feelings of hopelessness and unbearable psychic pain in those who are suicidal are the antithesis of terrorist acts, and mental disorders do not appear to be a feature of terrorists. In fact, some have specifically denied suicidal intent, as suicide is proscribed by their religion and the act simply results in a shorter path to heaven.

Suicide bombers have been considered as examples of altruistic suicide, but typically that does not involve the death of others, unless in a military setting such as the Japanese Kamikaze pilots of World War II. Group indoctrination may take place, and blind obedience to a cause or to charismatic leaders may be a factor in some vulnerable persons. Whether that vulnerability is of a clinical nature, being related to early developmental experiences, or whether it is more appropriately regarded as predominantly of a political/military nature is open to speculation. However, the recent reviews have concluded that such terrorists are essentially participants in a political/military environment.

This leads to the inevitable conclusion that the term 'suicide bombers' is inappropriate, and should be replaced by 'homicide bombers'. This more accurately describes the indiscriminate murder, with the death of the bomber being incidental, rather than suicidal.

13.6 **Are no-harm contracts of value?**

Some clinicians treating those who are suicidal take comfort in devising no-harm contracts. Typically these state that the person will not attempt or die by suicide, and that they will adopt different help-seeking behaviour if a crisis arises. However, there is no evidence that they are of value, although their popularity has probably arisen because suicide is so infrequent statistically that virtually any intervention could be considered as successful by the individual clinician.

The term 'contract' implies concern for legal obligation rather than clinical responsibility, but the use of no-harm contracts does not absolve a therapist from making a full and careful assessment, rather than simply relying on such a contract. It has been suggested that a commitment to treatment statement would be preferable, and that has elements of manual based therapy consistent with cognitive behavioural principles. However, although such a statement has validity in terms of being more theoretically based, it also has not been subjected to evaluation.

13.7 Has de-institutionalization contributed to suicide?

There have been reports from the late 1970s onward from a number of different countries to the effect that some suicides could be regarded as an unwanted effect of modern administrative practices, impacting upon some young persons who previously would have been hospitalized for extended periods of time.

In support of there being an association, it was found that between 1960 and 1995 mortality rates by suicide rose substantially in six countries in which bed numbers had decreased, whereas there had been a marginal decline in suicide in the only country, Japan, which had increased bed numbers during that time. It is also pertinent that the detailed UK Confidential Inquiry into suicide and homicide found that suicide was associated with a decrease in the provision of care, including being transferred to a less supervised setting at the last contact, and that was so even after controlling for previously perceived suicide risk.

Not only professional concern, but also public concern has been raised. From the historical point of view there has been comparison between the present state of patients with psychiatric illness being discharged to inadequate community care with the public outcry which led to changes in regard to the legal constraints about suicide in the early 19th century.

These observations are not made with a view to arguing for a return to the old mental hospital system, but, like all fashions, the pendulum has probably swung too far and good community residential care may be the most compassionate way forward for some of those who are chronically suicidal.

13.8 What is the role of the Internet in suicide prevention?

In a little over a decade the Internet has become a prime source of information about all aspects of health, as illustrated by an American survey which found that over half of an adult community sample, either personally or on behalf of another individual, had used the

Internet to cope with illness. Young people are more likely to use the Internet and they are twice as likely to go online rather than contacting a counselor or other health professional.

With specific regard to suicide, the Internet has been described as 'a double-edged tool'. On the one hand it can be used to source information about the means of suicide in a manner never before available, and it also provides a ready means of communication for like-minded suicidal persons. On the other hand, it can provide access not only to self-help programmes, but also to a range of helping agencies. Chat rooms are increasingly being used in place of tele-phone crisis lines, but whether that results in benefit or whether it reinforces suicidal behaviour is open to debate.

Internet programmes have been devised using cognitive behav-ioural principles to address symptoms of anxiety and depression. However, there are concerns about the lack of quality control criteria and supervision, although this has been addressed by the newly established International Society for Research into Internet Interven-tions. An Australian programme, MoodGym, has met the required standards and is effective in reducing symptoms of depression. Whether such interventions have an effect on suicidal behaviours per se remains to be determined, but it is inevitable that there will be increasing interest in research in this area.

13.9 Are enquiries about suicide useful?

This question applies not to specific research projects, but to *ad hoc* enquiries about individual suicides which may occur during the course of clinical practice. Naturally many will be subject to Coronial enquiry, but others will be investigated by local Hospital or Community Boards.

When suicide occurs the antecedents often appear in stark relief and it is sometimes compelling to conclude that various interventions should or should not have been undertaken, and that they would have influenced the outcome. Clinicians are not immune to such speculations, and inevitably alternative management scenarios can be envisaged. This often leads to self and team blame, and enquiries will be perceived as threatening.

In conducting an enquiry into suicide there are two broad questions which need to be addressed. The first and often most pressing from the point of view of administrators and those bereaved by the suicide is whether or not the suicide could have been predicted, with the presumed corollary that it could have been prevented. The answer to this question is almost invariably no, because although risk factors predict when aggregate data are considered, none of those so called risk factors either singly or in combination are reliable in predicting an individual suicide.

The second and more important question is whether or not management practices were within the realms of good practice. That is where an objective reviewer can be reassuring that appropriate management has occurred and that the suicide has been an unexpected outcome, notwithstanding the fact that treatment may have been optimal. On the other hand, if management practices are found wanting, comment should be made, albeit with the caveat that even if such management practices had been utilized, there could be no guarantee that the suicide would not have occurred.

Those entrusted with the onerous duty of participating in enquiries after suicide are aware of the need for tact in pointing out any shortcomings in management, as the suicide of a patient is particularly distressing. Inappropriately harsh criticisms can be destructive for both individual therapists and teams, particularly when there are systemic shortcomings which have placed high demands on staff. For an enquiry to be useful, clearly the focus needs to be on seeking areas that can be improved, rather than apportioning blame.

References

Appleby, L., Shaw, J., Amos, T., et al. (1999). Suicide within twelve months of contact with mental health services; national clinical survey. B.M.J., **318**, 1235–9.

Christensen, H., Griffiths, K. (2007). Reaching standards for dissemination: a case study. Med. Info., **12**. 459–63.

Crandall, C., Fullerton-Gleason, L., Aguero, R., La Valley, J. (2006). Subsequent suicide mortality among emergency department patients seen for suicidal behaviour. Acad. Emerg. Med., **13**, 435–42.

Goldney, R.D. (2003). De-institutionalisation and suicide. Crisis, **24**, 39–40.

Goodyer, I., Dubicka, B., Wilkinson, P. et al. (2007). Selective Serotonin Reuptake Inhibitors (SSRIs) and routine specialists care with and without cognitive behaviour therapy in adolescents with major depression: randomised controlled trial. B.M.J. **335**, 142–50.

Gould, M.S., Marrocco, F.A., Kleinman, M. et al. (2005). Evaluating iatrogenic risk of youth suicide screening programs: a randomized controlled trial. J.A.M.A., **293**, 1635–43.

MoodGym (2007). http://www.moodgym.anu.edu.au/

Pridmore, S., Ahmadi, J., Evenhuis, M. (2006). Suicide for scutinizers. Australas. Psychiat., **14**, 359–64.

Rudd, M.D., Mandrusiak, M., Joiner, T. (2007). The case against No-Suicide Contracts: The commitment to treatment statement as a practice alternative. J. Clin. Psychol.: In Session, **62**, 243–51.

Tam, J., Tang, W.S., Ferando, D.J. (2007). The Internet and suicide: a double-edged tool. *Eur. J. Intern. Med.*, **18**, 453–55.

Townsend, E. Suicide Terrorists: Are They Suicidal? Suicide and Life-Threatening Behavior, 2007, **37**, 35–49.

Whitlock, J., Lader, W., Conterio, K. (2007). The Internet and self-injury: what psychotherapists should know. *J. Clin. Psychol.*: In Session, **63**, 1135–43.

Chapter 14

Conclusion

> ### Key points
> - No single approach is suitable for all
> - A range of effective approaches is available which can be tailored to specific situations or individuals
> - It is important not to lose focus on the management of mental disorders in the individual suicidal person
> - There is no need to be pessimistic about our capacity to prevent suicide.

14.1 The knowledge base

It is no longer acceptable to state blandly that we do not know the relative importance of risk factors for suicide, or that there is no convincing evidence for the effectiveness of suicide prevention measures. It is unrealistic to expect a management approach to suit all, but there are a number of approaches which are effective and which can be adopted for different countries and different clinical populations.

A number of broad societal factors such as socio-economic and civil status are associated with suicide rates; access to high lethality means of suicide contributes to suicide; irresponsible media reporting is associated with increased suicide; longitudinal birth cohort case-controlled studies have identified and clarified the inter-relationship between early development risk factors and subsequent suicidal behaviour; twin studies have confirmed the importance of both inherited and environmental factors; it is now appreciated that there is a biology of suicidal behaviour; and detailed clinical studies have highlighted the importance of individual psychodynamics, and in particular perceived interpersonal rejection in precipitating the final act.

It is important to reiterate that population attributable risk research has placed various risk factors in perspective, and in developed countries the overwhelming importance of severe mental disorders has become apparent. This is to the extent that issues such as unemployment or poverty, whilst important in their own right and which should be addressed by appropriate social action, should be of little concern to the individual clinician. At the very least it is important that clinicians are not distracted by such issues, and that focus remains on the optimum management of those mental disorders which are more proximally associated with suicidal behaviours.

It is also evident that the gold standard of the RCT is unlikely to ever be a practical approach to demonstrating the effectiveness of specific interventions. Astute investors are aware that there are other precious metals beside gold, and experienced researchers are aware that there are innovative research methodologies other than RCTs which have demonstrated the effectiveness of a number of interventions.

It is sobering to reflect on research that has demonstrated that standard treatments do not appear to have been used in a significant proportion of those who die by suicide. That is consistent with findings from the UK and Australia that about 20% of suicides in association with hospitalization could have been preventable, but for poor staff-patient relationships, inadequate assessment and management of depression and other disorders, and poor continuity of care, particularly in the transition period between hospitalization and the community. In brief this means shortcomings in the provision of standard care. Therefore it is not unexpected that a study from the United States reported a strong correlation between suicide rates and indicators of access to health care, thereby emphasizing that clinical intervention was a crucial element in suicide prevention.

14.2 The way ahead

The way ahead is clear. Broad social services efforts to counteract childhood antecedents of suicidal behaviour are important in their own right and may pay dividends in terms of a reduction in suicide in the future. However, for more immediate results, a number of effective prevention of access to means of suicide programmes have been demonstrated, tailored to particular countries or sites; a focussed community approach such as the United States Air Force project is a model which could be emulated elsewhere; and, importantly for the clinician at the individual level, standard assessment and management practices for those with mental disorders should be implemented for all who are suicidal.

Not all clinicians should feel obliged to continue the management of patients who are suicidal. However, they should all possess the clinical skills to make a general assessment and management plan, albeit with a view to referral to a colleague with specific interest and expertise in the management of interpersonal problems for those without mental disorders, or to appropriate professionals when mental disorders are delineated. Whereas in the past there was a sense of pessimism about our capacity to prevent suicidal behaviour, now there is sound evidence for the effectiveness of standard treatments for mental disorders that are associated with suicidal behaviour.

Naturally not all suicide can be prevented: some persons will have intractable illnesses resistant to all interventions, and others will avoid assessment and management. However, by utilizing knowledge gained from two centuries of suicide prevention research, and by putting it into practice in a manner similar to the effective interventions described, there is every reason to believe that the unacceptable rate of suicide world wide can be reduced.

References

Burgess, P., Pirkis, J., Morton, J., Croke, E. (2000). Lessons from a comprehensive clinical audit of users of psychiatric services who committed suicide. *Psychiat. Serv.*, **51**, 1555–60.

Goldney, R.D. (2005). Suicide prevention: a pragmatic review of recent studies. *Crisis*, **26**, 128–40.

National Confidential Inquiry. (2001). Safety first: Five-year report of the National Confidential Inquiry into suicide and homicide by people with mental illness. London: Department of Health Publications.

Pitman, A. (2007). Policy on the prevention of suicidal behaviour; one treatment for all may be an unrealistic expectation. *J. R. Soc. Med.*, **100**, 461–4.

Sudden Unexplained Death (SUD) Study Collaborators. (2006). Avoidable deaths: five year report of the national confidential inquiry into suicide and homicide by people with mental illness. The University of Manchester.

Tondo, L., Albert, M.J., Baldessarini, R.J. (2005). Suicide rates in relation to health care access in the United States: an ecological study. *J. Clin. Psychiat.*, **67**, 517–23.

Useful links

International organizations

International Association for Suicide Prevention (IASP)

The IASP was founded in Vienna in 1960 and is a non-profit organization in official relationship with the World Health Organisation. Members from over 50 countries include researchers, clinicians, volunteers, and other professionals who share their knowledge and collaborate on suicide prevention world wide. International Congresses are held each two years, and regional conferences are also co-sponsored.

www.med.uio.no/iasp

Email: iasp1960@aol.com

Samaritans

The Samaritans was founded in 1953 in England and now has over 200 affiliated centres in 38 countries.

www.samaritans.org in UK and Ireland

www.befrienders.org elsewhere

Lifeline International

Lifeline International was established in 1963 in Australia, and now provides services in 15 countries, predominately in the Southern Hemisphere.

www.lifeline-international.org

International Federation of Telephone Emergency Services (IFOTES)

IFOTES has 20 full member countries and nine associated member country organizations, predominantly in Europe.

www.ifotes.org

International Academy of Suicide Research (IASR)

The IASR was established in 1990 as a forum to promote and disseminate research into suicidal behaviours.

www.iasronline.org

National suicide prevention organizations

American Association of Suicidology
www.suicidology.org

Email: info@suicidology.org

Canadian Association for Suicide Protection
www.casp-acps.ca

Email: admin@casp-acps.ca

Irish Association of Suicidology
www.ias.ie

Email: office@ias.ie

Suicide Prevention Australia
www.suicidepreventionaust.org

Email: info@suicidepreventionaust.org

Index